Advances in Urology®
Volume 4

Advances in Urology®

Volume 1

Volume 2

Advances in
Urology®

Editor-in-Chief
Bernard Lytton, M.B., F.R.C.S.

Professor and Chief, Section of Urology, Yale University School of Medicine,
New Haven, Connecticut

Editorial Board
William J. Catalona, M.D.

Professor and Chief, Division of Urologic Surgery, Department of Surgery,
Washington University School of Medicine, St. Louis, Missouri

Larry I. Lipshultz, M.D.

Professor of Urology, Department of Urology, Baylor College of Medicine,
Houston, Texas

Edward J. McGuire, M.D.

Professor and Head, Section of Urology, University of Michigan, University
Hospitals, Ann Arbor, Michigan

Volume 4 · 1991

Mosby
Year Book

St. Louis   Baltimore   Boston   Chicago   London   Philadelphia   Sydney   Toronto

KCUM Dept. of Surgery

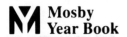
**Mosby
Year Book**

Dedicated to Publishing Excellence

Sponsoring Editor: Amy L. Zekas
Associate Managing Editor, Manuscript Services: Denise Dungey
Assistant Director, Manuscript Services: Frances M. Perveiler
Production Coordinator: Max Perez
Proofroom Manager: Barbara M. Kelly

Editorial Office:
Mosby–Year Book, Inc.
200 North LaSalle St.
Chicago, IL 60601

International Standard Serial Number: 0894-4385
International Standard Book Number: 0-8151-5692-8

Contributors

Henry R. Black, M.D.
Professor of Internal Medicine, Director, Preventive Cardiology Service, Yale University School of Medicine, New Haven, Connecticut

David A. Bloom, M.D.
Associate Professor of Surgery, University of Michigan Medical School; Chief, Pediatric Urology, Mott Children's Hospital, Ann Arbor, Michigan

Bruce Blyth, M.D., F.R.A.C.S.
Lecturer in Surgery/Urology, University of Pennsylvania School of Medicine; Attending Urologist, Children's Hospital of Philadelphia, Philadelphia, Pennsylvania

Fredric L. Coe, M.D.
University of Chicago, Pritzker School of Medicine, Nephrology Program, Chicago, Illinois

Lester A. Klein, M.D.
Urologist, Scripps Clinic and Research Institute, La Jolla, California

Donald L. Lamm, M.D.
Professor and Chairman, Department of Urology, West Virginia University School of Medicine, West Virginia University Medical Center, Morgantown, West Virginia

Terrence R. Malloy, M.D.
Professor of Urology, University of Pennsylvania School of Medicine, Philadelphia, Pennsylvania

James E. Montie, M.D.
Chairman, Department of Urology, Cleveland Clinic Florida, Fort Lauderdale, Florida

Pat D. O'Donnell, M.D.
Professor, Department of Urology, University of Arkansas for Medical Sciences, College of Medicine; Director, Arkansas Center for Incontinence; Chief, Little Rock Veterans Administration Medical Center; Little Rock, Arkansas

Angelo S. Paola, M.D.
Resident in Urology, West Virginia University School of Medicine, West Virginia University Medical Center, Morgantown, West Virginia

Joan Parks, M.B.A.
University of Chicago, Pritzker School of Medicine, Nephrology Program, Chicago, Illinois

Carol M. Proudfit, Ph.D.

Assistant Division Director, Division of Drugs and Toxicology, American Medical Association, Chicago, Illinois

Claus G. Röhrborn, M.D.

Division of Urology, Southwestern Medical School, University of Texas Southwestern Medical Center at Dallas, Dallas, Texas

Mark C. Saddler, M.B.Ch.B.

Westchester County Foundation, Fellow in Hypertension, Yale University School of Medicine, New Haven, Connecticut

Fritz H. Schröder, M.D.

Professor and Chairman, Department of Urology, Erasmus University, Rotterdam, The Netherlands

Kurt Semm, o. Prof. Dr. Med. Dr. Med. Vet h.c.

Direktor der Abteilung Frauenheilkunde im Klinikum der Christian-Albrechts-Universität, Kiel, Germany

Preface

The fourth volume of *Advances in Urology* provides an updated review of several common urological problems. Included are discussions of some of the newer methods being used in the treatment of BPH and the role of laparoscopy in the management of intra-abdominal testes in children.

Drs. Lamm and Paola provide an excellent review on the use of BCG in the treatment of superficial tumors and carcinoma in situ of the bladder. A complete response rate is now seen in 70%–80% of patients treated with BCG. They also describe some new agents that are presently being developed for intravesical immunotherapy. Invasive bladder cancer is still one of the most challenging problems for the urologist. Dr. Montie has written a very thoughtful and up-to-date review of the managment of this disease that includes surgery, the latest forms of diversion, and alternative methods of treatment that are aimed at sparing the bladder.

There have been a number of interesting new advances in the endocrine management of prostatic cancer in recent years. These have led to some controversy and a change in the way patients are managed by hormonal manipulation. Drs. Schröder and Röhrborn have written a scholarly and informative review of this subject and clearly analyze the basis of some of the controversies that have arisen.

New methods of removing tissue endoscopically have been developed and Dr. Malloy describes his experience with cavitron aspiration of the prostate. This can be done more quickly and with less bleeding than the standard procedure. The method has also been used elsewhere for endoscopic removal of solid organs and may well become an established procedure in the near future. Balloon dilatation of the prostate remains a controversial technique for the treatment of benign prostatic hypertrophy. Dr. Klein, one of the early and enthusiastic proponents of this method, has written an excellent account of his experience. Dr. Proudfit of the Division of Drugs and Toxicology of the American Medical Association gives a comprehensive and informative review of the current use of drugs and hormones in the management of disorders of the male reproductive system, providing a different perspective for the practicing urologist.

The medical management of stone disease is still an extremely important subject with which the urologist must remain familiar, despite the advent of the many new methods for the destruction of urinary calculi. Prevention is still preferred. Dr. Coe, a recognized authority on stone disease, and his assistant, Joan Parks, have written a review of their current approach to the metabolic problems of stone disease.

Incontinence in the elderly has become a major problem for the urologist. Dr. O'Donnell summarizes this very well and stresses the need to determine the etiology of incontinence in these patients so that it can be managed appropriately. A correctable renal problem is present in up to

10% of patients with hypertension. Angioplasty and corrective renal surgery are still important alternatives or adjuncts to drug therapy in many cases. Drs. Black and Saddler, who have considerable experience derived from the hypertensive study group at Yale, have written a very clear and comprehensive account of the diagnosis and management of renal hypertension. Endoscopic management of intra-abdominal problems is becoming increasingly popular. Laparoscopy in patients with undescended impalpable testes has greatly enhanced the management of this condition. Endoscopic orchiectomy and preliminary clipping of the vessels is now becoming more widely practiced, and the article by Drs. Bloom & Semm should stimulate adoption of these methods by the practicing urologist.

The last chapter by Dr. Bruce Blyth of Children's Hospital of Philadelphia is an excellent review of the current management of ambiguous genitalia in children, and should provide a ready reference for any urologist who may suddenly be presented with this problem.

Bernard Lytton, M.B., F.R.C.S.

Contents

Bacillus Calmette-Guerin Immunotherapy in Bladder Cancer

Angelo S. Paola, M.D.

Resident in Urology, West Virginia University School of Medicine, West Virginia University Medical Center, Morgantown, West Virginia

Donald L. Lamm, M.D.

Professor and Chairman, Department of Urology, West Virginia University School of Medicine, West Virginia University Medical Center, Morgantown, West Virginia

Bladder cancer is the sixth leading malignancy in the United States, responsible for an estimated 49,000 new cases and 9,700 deaths each year.[1] It continues to have a male predominance (3:1), and whites are affected more commonly than blacks by a 4:1 ratio.[2] Histologically, transitional cell carcinoma accounts for 90% of the cases, squamous cell carcinoma for 8%, and adenocarcinoma for approximately 2%.[2] Superficial transitional cell carcinoma, i.e., tumor confined to the mucosa (Ta or Tcis) or with invasion of the lamina propria (T1), accounts for approximately 80% of all cases at presentation.[3] Up to 80% of patients treated by initial endoscopic resection of superficial disease will experience tumor recurrence, and as many as 30% of these will progress to muscle invasive disease.[4] Factors that increase the risk of tumor recurrence include urothelial dysplasia, carcinoma in situ, lamina propria invasion, tumor multiplicity, rapid recurrence, size >3 cm, and higher grade (II or III).[5]

Intravesical therapy has been designed to eradicate residual tumor if present (treatment) and to delay or prevent subsequent recurrences (prophylaxis). In recent years, the immunotherapy of bladder cancer has gained increasing popularity. Immunotherapies are divided into two categories: active, in which administered immunostimulants induce the host's immune system to respond to tumor antigens; and passive, which transfers immunologically active reagents (serum, cells, or cell products) directly to the host in an attempt to mediate an antitumor response. Each of these groups can be separated further into specific and nonspecific immunostimulants based on their mechanisms of action.[6]

Bacillus Calmette-Guerin (BCG) thus far has proven to be the most successful form of immunotherapy for human malignancy, especially in the treatment of superficial bladder cancer. In this chapter, we will review the current knowledge regarding various aspects of BCG and its use, and then will discuss briefly some of the alternative forms of immunotherapy presently under investigation.

Historical Background

BCG was isolated by Auguste Calmette and Claude Guerin through progressive attenuation of a virulent strain of *Mycobacterium bovis*.[7] The first clinical use of this vaccine was in 1921 when oral BCG was used successfully to protect a girl born into a household where active tuberculosis infection was present.[7] Since that time, more than 1.5 billion BCG vaccinations have been performed with minimal morbidity and mortality.[8]

In the 4 decades after the application of BCG in tuberculosis prophylaxis, Freund and other immunologists discovered its remarkable stimulatory effect on the immune response, and in 1959 investigators began to evaluate it in the inhibition of tumor growth in animal models.[9, 10] Successful treatment of many animal tumors with BCG led to multiple clinical trials with human malignancies, including lung carcinoma, acute lymphocytic leukemia, acute and chronic myelocytic leukemia, breast carcinoma, ovarian carcinoma, renal carcinoma, carcinoma of the prostate, and non-Hodgkin's lymphoma.[11] In 1976, Morales reported the first clinical trial of intravesical BCG.[12] Richman et al. have demonstrated a therapeutic effect of intracavitary BCG on both pleural and peritoneal malignant effusions.[13] Recently, a significant increase in disease-free and overall survival was demonstrated in patients with non-Hodgkin's malignant lymphoma treated with adjuvant percutanous BCG.[14] However, the favorable results obtained by these and several other investigators using BCG to treat neoplasms other than transitional cell carcinoma have been sporadic, and only human bladder cancer has manifested a consistent, significant therapeutic benefit from this form of immunotherapy.[11]

Mechanism of Action

While BCG's efficacy cannot be denied, its specific mechanism of action in cancer immunotherapy is still largely unknown. BCG has been shown to be a potent immune adjuvant that heightens responses to antigenic stimulation.[15] These responses have included enhancement of both cell mediated and humoral immunity.

Although BCG administration results in an intense inflammatory cell infiltration of the bladder, the multiplicity of responses to BCG, as well as the observation that other inflammatory agents promote rather than inhibit bladder tumor growth, make it unlikely that nonspecific inflammation is the sole mechanism of action. The array of responses to BCG suggests that it affects a wide range of cell types including B cells, T cells, macrophages, killer (K) cells, and natural killer (NK) cells.[16] Elevations of interferon and interleukin-2 levels also have been noted with BCG therapy.[17, 18] The induction of cytotoxic T cell immunity is clearly one of the important mechanisms of action of BCG as evidenced by the fact that transfer of such cells in animals results in transfer of BCG-induced tumor protection.[19] Despite much research into this area, the complexity of immune responses to BCG continues to suggest that multiple factors are responsible for its antitumor effect; therefore, BCG continues to be looked upon as a potent nonspecific immunostimulant.[9]

Animal Studies

Experimental results with animal tumor models cannot be translated directly to the clinic; however, the experience gained from such experimentation can facilitate significantly the design of clinical protocols and expedite the delivery of therapeutic improvements. Studies with mouse models have suggested that BCG has decreased effectiveness when the tumor burden exceeds 100,000 cells. As a result, even though BCG has been remarkably effective in the treatment of patients with residual bladder cancer, every effort should be made to resect *all* tumor prior to initiating BCG immunotherapy.

An adequate number of viable BCG organisms is an essential requirement for successful BCG immunotherapy. Excessive BCG administration, or the use of nonviable preparations, can reduce the efficacy. In general, 1 $\times$ 10^7 organisms are required. Other factors that have been found to effect a favorable response to BCG include close proximity of BCG and tumor cells, an immune-competent host, and the presence of an antigenic tumor. All of these apply to transitional cell carcinoma of the urothelium.[10, 20]

The immunity induced by BCG has been observed to protect from subsequent tumor challenge for as long as 8 months without additional BCG treatment and as long as 15 months if additional BCG is given at the time of tumor inoculation.[21] Animal data continue to confirm that appropriate doses of local and/or systemic BCG inhibit the growth of transitional cell carcinoma. As will be seen later in this chapter, multiple other nonspecific immunotherapeutic agents including keyhole-limpet hemocyanin (KLH), levamisole, interferon, and interferon inducers have been shown to be effective in animal studies.

Clinical Trials

Since 1976 when Morales first reported a 12-fold reduction of tumor recurrence in nine patients treated with intravesical and percutaneous BCG, the significant advantage of BCG immunotherapy in preventing tumor recurrence has been confirmed by numerous clinical trials.[12] In a prospective randomized trial of transurethral resection alone or with intravesical BCG, Lamm et al. reported that tumor recurrence was decreased from 47.5% to 18.5% with the addition of intravesical BCG, and the mean disease-free interval was prolonged from 31 months to 58 months with BCG treatment.[22] A similar study at Memorial Sloan-Kettering Cancer Center reported a dramatic reduction in tumor recurrence from 2.37 tumors per patient month in controls to 0.7 tumors per patient month in the BCG group.[23] These results were confirmed by a follow-up study evaluating the long-term effects of BCG in the same treatment group.[24] Similar protection from tumor recurrence has been reported by numerous other investigators.[25-31] Dramatic reductions in tumor progression also have been reported with BCG as compared to surgery alone, with overall progression being reduced from 95% to 53%, progression to stage T2 reduced from 46% to 28%, cystectomy reduced from 42% to 25%, and deaths reduced from 32% to 14%.[32] Pagano has confirmed that BCG significantly reduces progression. In a randomized study, 18% of all patients had progression to stage T2 or higher compared with only 4% of those treated with BCG.[33]

Only two studies have failed to demonstrate any added benefit from BCG immunotherapy. Flamm and Grof observed a 59% recurrence rate in patients treated with intravesical Connaught strain BCG.[34] Stober and Peters compared transurethral surgery alone with surgery and percutaneous BCG and found no improved results with percutaneous BCG.[35] These studies suggest that the route of administration is an important consideration, especially when lower vaccine doses or shorter courses of therapy are used. Despite animal studies showing that BCG is rarely effective when tumor burden exceeds 100,000 cells, BCG has been very successful in treating patients with residual bladder cancer. Complete response rates have ranged from 36% to 83%, with a mean of 58%, and compare favorably with those for intravesical chemotherapy.[36] While this complete response rate is encouraging, it must be emphasized that every effort should be made to resect all tumor prior to initiating BCG immunotherapy.

Bacillus Calmette-Guerin in Carcinoma In Situ

The excellent complete response rate of carcinoma in situ to BCG treatment and the durability of these responses suggest that BCG is the treatment of choice for carcinoma in situ of the bladder. Several factors may account for the favorable responses observed in carcinoma in situ: (1) it is poorly differentiated and, presumably, very antigenic; (2) it involves only a few cell layers and tumor volume is small despite the presence of diffuse disease; and (3) it is very accessible to direct contact with BCG when confined to the bladder.

Reported response rates have ranged from 68% to 82%. The complete response rate of 74% noted in a combined experience using various substrains of BCG is higher than that reported with any other intravesical agent.[6] In an ongoing Southwest Oncology Group trial, 71% of patients randomized to BCG have had a complete response compared to 47% of patients treated with doxorubicin (Adriamycin), which, prior to BCG, has had the highest response rate in carcinoma in situ.[37] In 150 randomized

Southwest Oncology Group patients with carcinoma in situ, an additional three weekly BCG instillations given at 3 months increased the complete response rate from 70% to an impressive 82% ($P <.05$).[38]

As a result of the excellent and durable response rates of carcinoma in situ to BCG treatments, radical cystectomy is no longer the initial treatment of choice for this group of patients. Early cystectomy previously had been recommended for diffuse carcinoma in situ with concurrent multiple, superficial papillary tumors due to the high risk of progression to muscle-invasive disease (40% to 80% of cases within 5 years).[39] Review of our data on BCG treatment in high-risk patients, including patients with carcinoma in situ, revealed a significantly decreased risk of progression to muscle invasion compared to untreated controls.[40]

The vast majority of patients who do not respond completely to BCG will fail with localized disease that can be detected easily and treated effectively. Cystectomy is associated with significant morbidity and mortality, and there is no evidence from controlled studies to suggest that early cystectomy will increase overall survival or decrease morbidity. Therefore, we reserve cystectomy for those carcinoma in situ patients who fail BCG treatment.

Bacillus Calmette-Guerin in Muscle-Invasive Disease

The use of BCG in the treatment of muscle-invasive disease remains a controversial issue. In general, nonspecific immunotherapy with BCG or any other agent is felt to be ineffective in patients with significant tumor burden or invasive or metastatic disease. However, several documented responses have been noted with BCG treatment in patients with residual muscle-invasive tumor. It should be stressed that only patients who refused cystectomy or had a medical contraindication to radical surgery have been offered the alternative of BCG treatment.

Bacillus Calmette-Guerin Immunotherapy vs. Chemotherapy

Due to the fact that BCG's mechanism of action is different from that of the chemotherapeutic agents, cross-resistance is unlikely and has not been identified. Therefore, patients who have failed intravesical chemotherapy often will respond to BCG, and vice versa.[40]

BCG has been shown to be more effective than thiotepa in preventing tumor recurrence. Brosman reported a 47% recurrence rate in patients treated with thiotepa compared to 0% in the BCG treatment group.[26] In a preliminary evaluation of BCG-RIVM (Rijksinstituut voor Volksgezondheid en Milieuhygiene) compared with mitomycin C, no advantage of either agent was apparent.[41] However, concern has been raised about the efficacy of the RIVM preparation, and a subsequent comparison of Pasteur BCG and mitomycin C found BCG to be superior.

A prospective study recently completed by the Southwest Oncology Group has demonstrated BCG immunotherapy to be superior to doxorubicin chemotherapy.[37] Complete resolution of carcinoma in situ occurred in 72% of BCG-treated patients but in only 46% of doxorubicin-treated patients. BCG also significantly reduced the recurrence rate for papillary tumors: 26% in the BCG group compared to 40% in the doxorubicin-treated patients.[37]

Martinez-Pineiro et al. recently reported their data from a randomized prospective trial involving 202 patients comparing the prophylactic effect of 15 courses of 50 mg of doxorubicin, 50 mg of thiotepa, or 150 mg of Pasteur BCG instilled intravesically against recurrences and progression of superficial transitional cell bladder cancer.[42] The number of recurrences was significantly lower in the BCG arm (13.4%) compared to the thioteta (35.7%) and doxorubicin (43.4%) arms. The overall progression rate for BCG-treated patients was 1.5%, significantly lower than that of the patients treated with thiotepa (3.6%) or doxorubicin (7.5%).

Despite a long and extensive experience with multiple intravesical chemotherapies, there is no strong evidence that this form of treatment reduces the incidence of muscle invasion, tumor progression, or long-term recurrence rate, or that it improves patient survival.[6] On the other hand, as stated earlier, BCG has led to dramatic reductions in tumor progression and to improvements in patient survival.[32] The higher response rates to BCG and the low incidence of significant complications have led us to use this agent as the primary treatment of choice for superficial transitional cell carcinoma of the bladder.

Bacillus Calmette-Guerin Dosage and Administration

The initial endoscopic evaluation of the patient with transitional cell carcinoma of the bladder is important in designing the subsequent treatment plan, which will depend on the stage and grade of the resected tumor as well as other risk factors for recurrent disease. For example, a patient who has a grade I stage Ta tumor, no prior history of tumor, and a normal cytology following resection would not be a candidate for intravesical therapy. On the other hand, patients with tumors larger than 3 cm in diameter, multiple tumors, grade II–III histology, lamina propria invasion, recurrent tumor, or carcinoma in situ will require intravesical therapy.

The optimal protocol for BCG immunotherapy remains undefined. Preparations of BCG that have been demonstrated to be effective intravesically include Armand-Frappier, BCG-RIVM, Connaught, Evans (Glaxo), Pasteur, Japanese, and Tice. Although optimal doses have not been established, commonly used effective intravesical doses are 120 mg for Armand-Frappier, RIVM, and Connaught; 75 to 150 mg for Pasteur; 50 mg for Tice; and 40 mg for Japanese BCG. In the United States, the Connaught and Tice preparations are commercially available.[6]

Therapy is usually initiated within 2 weeks of tumor resection to provide optimal juxtaposition of BCG and any residual tumor as well as to stimulate a strong immune response.[20] Treatments should be delayed 1 to 2 weeks after extensive resections to decrease the risk of absorption and sepsis. Although the necessity of maintenance immunotherapy is still debatable, increasing evidence suggests that a single 6-week course of BCG, though highly effective, is suboptimal for many patients.[30, 43] Preliminary review of our Southwest Oncology Group data has demonstrated that an additional 3-week course of intravesical BCG 3 months after the initiation of therapy can increase the complete response rates significantly when compared to a single 6-week course (82% vs. 70% complete response, respectively).[38] Neither percutaneous nor oral BCG administration has been shown to improve antitumor response over intravesical therapy alone; therefore, we feel that intravesical instillation alone is sufficient.[44, 45]

The decision to give maintenance BCG treatments might be based on patient risk factors, since it is unlikely that all patients will require it. It is important to note that some patients will require more than a single 6-week course of treatment to prevent tumor recurrence or to eradicate carcinoma in situ completely.[23, 26, 43] This suggests that a patient should not be considered to have failed BCG therapy unless he has had at least two 6-week courses of BCG or has developed progressive disease while on treatment. It should be stressed, however, that high-risk patients should not continue on ineffective intravesical therapy while the disease progresses beyond the limit of surgical excision.

TABLE 1.
Bacillus Calmette-Guerin Doses and Treatment Schedules

Treatment schedules

Morales: Intravesically and percutaneously weekly for 6 weeks.
Brosman: Intravesically weekly for 6 weeks, then monthly.
Lamm: First course—intravesically weekly for 6 weeks, then weekly for three instillations at 3 months, then at 6 months, then every 6 months for up to 4 years. Second course—intravesically weekly for 2 weeks, every other week for three treatments, monthly for 4 months, and then every 6 months for 4 years.

Effective vaccine doses

Armand-Frappier: 120 mg
Connaught: 120 mg
Pasteur: 75–150 mg
Tice: 50 mg
Japanese: 40 mg

Based on the above information and our own experience, we would recommend 50 mg of Tice BCG (1 ampule) or 120 mg of Connaught (3 ampules) in 50 ml of normal saline weekly for a 6-week course, then weekly for 3 weeks at 3 months, with subsequent single treatments at 6 months, and every 6 months thereafter for up to 4 years (first course). Many patients who have recurrence of tumor after BCG will respond to another course given as follows: weekly for 2 weeks, then every other week for three treatments, then monthly for 4 months, then every 6 months for up to 4 years (second course). Other treatment schedules reported can be found in Table 1.[6]

Complications of Intravesical Bacillus Calmette-Guerin Therapy

The superiority of BCG immunotherapy for the treatment and prophylaxis of superficial bladder cancer has led to its increased use throughout the world. As a result, the number and variety of complications observed to occur from this treatment has increased also. The major complications have been reviewed recently (Table 2).[46] Life-threatening and even fatal complications of BCG therapy have been reported.[46, 47] These are rare, however, and most patients tolerate therapy well.

The most common side effect noted with intravesical BCG, occurring in approximately 91% of patients, is granulomatous cystitis with irritative voiding symptoms of frequency and dysuria. Symptoms usually begin after the second or third instillation and persist for about 2 days. Phenazopyridine (Pyridium) (200 mg) and oxybutynin (Ditropan) (5 mg) orally three times daily have been useful in minimizing these symptoms. For severe irritative symptoms, 300 mg of oral isoniazid taken the day before treatment and for 2 days afterward has reduced patient discomfort. Mild gross hematuria has been noted, and approximately 25% of patients will experience constitutional symptoms such as low-grade fever, malaise, or nausea. Fever of greater than 103° F (39.5° C) has been reported in 2.9% of patients, and it usually resolves in 1 to 2 days with antipyretics and fluids. However, since patients with an uncomplicated febrile response cannot be distinguished from those who will develop systemic BCG infection, they should be hospitalized and treated with antituberculous medications.[46] Granulomatous prostatitis has been noted in 1.3% of patients treated and cannot be distinguished from carcinoma of the prostate without a biopsy specimen.

Systemic BCG infection involving the lungs or liver has occurred in approximately 1% of patients. This usually responds to isoniazid and rifampin; however, in cases of acute septic or anaphylactic shock, cycloserine and prednisone should be added to the usual antituberculous regimen. Cycloserine has been shown to inhibit BCG growth within 1 day, while isoniazid and other antibiotics take up to 1 week to act. Also, since a cell-mediated immune response may contribute to the cause of shock, cor-

TABLE 2.
Complications of Bacillus
Calmette-Guerin Therapy

Type	Percent
Cystitis	91
Constitutional symptoms (malaise, nausea)	25
Fever (>39.5° C)	2.9
Hematuria	1.0
Granulomatous prostatitis	0.9
Pneumonitis/hepatitis	0.7
Arthralgia	0.5
Epididymo-orchitis	0.4
Sepsis	0.4
Rash	0.3
Ureteral obstruction	0.3
Contracted bladder	0.2
Cytopenia	0.1
Renal abscess	0.1

ticosteroids may be helpful. Unpublished research from our laboratory clearly demonstrates that septic deaths in mice given high-dose intraperitoneal BCG are in part related to hypersensitivity, and that survival is improved significantly with prednisone treatment. Intraperitoneal doses of BCG that are uniformly tolerated by unimmunized mice are uniformly fatal in immunized mice. Survival to BCG challenge is increased significantly in sensitized mice with the use of isoniazid, rifampin, and cycloserine, but not isoniazid, rifampin, and ethambutol. The highest survival (80%) was observed consistently in mice treated with isoniazid, rifampin, and prednisone. In cases of life-threatening infections, therefore, we suggest 250 to 500 mg of cycloserine twice daily and 40 mg of prednisone (or its equivalent) daily in addition to isoniazid and rifampin. Patients with severe symptoms should be treated subsequently with intravesical chemotherapy rather than BCG.

Other rare complications of BCG therapy have included arthalgia (.5%), skin rash (.3%), epididymo-orchitis (.4%), ureteral obstruction (.3%), bladder contracture (.2%), renal abscess (.1%), and pancytopenia (.1%). Immune-complex glomerulonephritis, choroiditis, nephrogenic adenoma, cardiac toxicity secondary to high fevers, pelvic abscess due to BCG extravasation after bladder perforation, and induction or promotion of tumor growth all have been reported, but occur so infrequently that incidences cannot be estimated.[46]

Comparison of toxicity between BCG and intravesical chemotherapeutic agents reveals that local toxicity is seen more frequently with BCG than with the commonly used chemotherapeutic agents.[46] Also, the overall number of side effects has been shown to be slightly higher in patients receiving BCG than in those treated with intravesical chemotherapy.[46] While the side effects and complications of BCG should not be minimized, it is important to note that the benefits of this therapy far exceed its risks, and that the vast majority of patients have no significant side effects.

Alternative Forms of Immunotherapy

BCG is currently the most effective intravesical therapy available for superficial bladder cancer. However, in patients with rapidly recurrent disease, as many as 57% will have tumor recurrence.[3] The number of patients who have failed BCG, in addition to its aforementioned toxicity, indicate the need for more effective and even less toxic forms of therapy. The demonstrated immunosensitivity of bladder cancer has led to the study of other immunostimulants, many of which have been used successfully in animal models and even in recent human trials.[6]

Keyhole-limpet hemocyanin is a complex protein found in the marine mollusk *Megathura crenulata,* and is one of the most immunogenic of antigens.[48] Olsson was the first to report a marked reduction in tumor recurrence in patients immunized with subcutaneous keyhole-limpet hemocyanin.[49] Dosages for this agent have ranged from 10 to 30 mg in an equal volume of normal saline given intravesically with a 1-mg intradermal injection weekly for 4 weeks and then monthly.[6]

Jurincic et al. found keyhole-limpet hemocyanin to be superior to mitomycin C, and Flamm reported it to be equal to triethylene glycol diglycerol ether (Epodyl) in preventing tumor recurrence.[50, 51] Therefore, it is potentially more effective than BCG. No toxicity has been reported to occur with keyhole-limpet hemocyanin; however, further controlled studies will have to be performed before its beneficial effects can be firmly established.

Several other agents currently are being investigated for their ability to selectively enhance the body's immune response. These include various lymphokines such as interferon, interleukin-2, and tumor necrosis factor; monoclonal antibodies; lymphokine-activated killer cells; maltose tetrapalmitate; poly inosinic polycytidylic acid (poly I:C); irradiated tumor vaccine; bropirimine; and butanol-extracted antigen.[6] All of these have been shown to have some antitumor activity, and although controlled studies presently are being conducted to confirm their effectiveness, the preliminary results with many of these treatments have been promising.

Conclusion

In recent decades, immunotherapy has been added to the armamentarium in the treatment of bladder cancer. BCG has been shown to reduce the incidence of tumor recurrence and progression significantly when compared to no treatment or chemotherapy. Due to the high complete response rates (74%) in carcinoma in situ, BCG has changed our management of this disease significantly. Recent approval by the Food and Drug Administration of BCG for the treatment of superficial bladder cancer will allow an even greater experience with its use; however, to date, evidence has proven that BCG is both highly effective and safe in the management of transitional cell carcinoma. Promising new immunotherapeutic agents, such as keyhole-limpet hemocyanin, vaccines, interleukin-2, and other lymphokines will be welcome additions to the clinical armamentarium, since they hold the promise of increased efficacy with reduced toxicity.

References

1. Silverberg E, Boring CC, Squires TS: Cancer statistics, 1990. *Ca* 1990; 40:9.
2. Droller MJ: Transitional cell cancer: Upper tracts and bladder, in Walsh PC, Gittes RF, Perlmutter AD, et al: (eds): *Campbell's Urology*, ed 5. Philadelphia, WB Saunders, 1986, p 1343.
3. Kowalkowski TS, Lamm DL: Intravesical therapy of superficial bladder cancer, in Resnick M (ed): *Current Trends in Urology*, vol 4. Baltimore, Williams & Wilkins Co, 1988, p 94.
4. Soloway MS: Diagnosis and management of superficial bladder cancer. *Semin Surg Oncol* 1989; 5:247–256.
5. Heney NM, Ahmed S, Flanagan MJ, et al: Superficial bladder cancer: Progression and recurrence. *J Urol* 1983; 130:1083.
6. Sosnowski JT, Lamm DL: Immunotherapy of bladder cancer. *Urology Annual* 1990; 4:123.
7. Crispen RG: BCG vaccine in perspective. *Semin Oncol* 1974; 1:311.
8. Lotte A, Wafz-Hockert O, Poisson N, et al: BCG complication: Estimated risks among vaccinated subjects and statistical analysis of the main characteristics. *Advances in Tuberculosis Research* 1984; 21:107.
9. Freund J: The mode of action of immunologic adjuvants. *Advances in Tuberculosis Research* 1956; 7:130.
10. Bast RC Jr, Zbar D, Borsos T, et al: BCG and cancer. *N Engl J Med* 1974; 290:1413.
11. Terry WD, Rosenberg SA (eds): *Immunotherapy of Human Cancer*. New York, Elsevier North-Holland Inc, 1981.
12. Morales A, Eidenger D, Bruce AW: Intracavity bacillus Calmette-Guerin in treatment of superficial bladder tumors. *J Urol* 1976; 116:180.
13. Richman SP, Hersh EM, Gutterman JU, et al: Administration of BCG cell wall skeleton into malignant effusions: Toxic and therapeutic effects. *Cancer Treatment Reports* 1981; 65:383.
14. Ravaud A, Eghbali H, Trojani M, et al: Adjuvant bacillus Calmette-Guerin therapy in non-Hodgkin's malignant lymphomas: Long term results of a randomized trial in a single institution. *J Clin Oncol* 1990; 8:608.
15. Winters WD, Lamm DL: Antibody responses to bacillus Calmette-Guerin immunotherapy in bladder cancer patients. *Cancer Res* 1981; 41:2672.
16. Davies M: Bacillus Calmette-Guerin as an anti-tumor agent. The interaction

with cells of the mammalian immune system. *Biochim Biophys Acta 1982; 651:143.*

17. Winters WD, Lamm DL: BCG-induced circulating interferon, antibody, and immune complexes in bladder cancer patients treated with intravesical BCG. *J Urol 1985; 134:40.*

18. Haaf ED, Catalona WJ, Ratliffe TL: Detection of interleukin-2 in urine of patients with superficial bladder tumors after treatment with intravesical BCG. *J Urol 1986; 136:970.*

19. Davies M, Sabbadini E: Mechanisms of BCG action: *Cancer Immunol Immunother 1982; 14:46.*

20. Lamm DL: BCG immunotherapy for superficial bladder cancer, in Ratliff TL, Catalona WJ (eds): *Genitourinary Cancer.* Boston, Martinus Nijhoff Publishers, 1987, p 205.

21. Reichert DF, Lamm DL: Long term protection in bladder cancer following intralesional immunotherapy. *J Urol 1984; 132:570.*

22. Lamm DL, Thor DE, Harris SC, et al: Bacillus Calmette-Guerin immunotherapy of superficial bladder cancer. *J Urol 1980; 124:38.*

23. Camacho F, Pinsky CM, Kerr D, et al: Treatment of superficial bladder cancer with intravesical BCG, in Terry WT, Rosenburg SA (eds): *The Immunotherapy of Cancer.* New York, Elsevier North-Holland, 1982, p 309.

24. Sarosdy MF, Lamm DL: Long term results of intravesical bacillus Calmette-Guerin therapy for superficial bladder cancer. *J Urol 1989; 142:719.*

25. Martinez-Peneiro JA: BCG vaccine in the treatment of non-infiltrating papillary tumors of the bladder, in Pavone-Macabew M, Smith PH, Edsmyr F (eds): *Bladder Tumors and Other Topics in Urologic Oncology.* New York, Plenum Press, 1980, p 173.

26. Brosman SA: Experience with bacillus Calmette-Guerin in patients with superficial bladder cancer. *J Urol 1982; 128:27.*

27. Adolphs HD, Bastian HP: Chemoimmune prophylaxis of superficial bladder tumors. *J Urol 1983; 129:29.*

28. Babayan RK, Krone RS: Intravesical BCG for superficial bladder cancer. Presented at the 80th annual meeting of the American Urologic Association, Atlanta, Georgia, May 1985.

29. deKernion JB, Huang MY, Linder A, et al: The management of superficial bladder tumors and carcinoma in situ with intravesical bacillus Calmette-Guerin. *J Urol 1985; 133:598.*

30. Haaf ED, Kelly DR, Dressner SN, et al: Results of retreatment with intravesical BCG therapy for patients failing the initial BCG course. Presented at the 80th annual meeting of the American Urologic Association, Atlanta, Georgia, May 1985.

31. Schellhammer PF, Ladaga LE: Bacillus Calmette-Guerin for therapy of superficial transitional cell carcinoma of the bladder. *J Urol 1986; 135:261.*

32. Herr HW, Laudone VP, Badalament RA: Bacillus Calmette-Guerin (BCG) therapy alters progression of superficial bladder cancer. *J Urol 1988; 139:229A.*

33. Pagano F, Bassi P, Milani C, et al: Effectiveness of low dose (75 mg) bacillus Calmette-Guerin therapy in superficial bladder cancer. Presented at American Urologic Association Annual Meeting, Dallas, Texas, May 1989.

34. Flamm J, Grof F: Adjuvant local immunotherapy with bacillus Calmette-Guerin (BCG) in treatment of urothelial carcinoma of the urinary bladder. *Wien Med Wochenschr 1981; 131:501.*

35. Stober U, Peters HH: BCG-immunotherapie zur rezidiuphylaxe bein harnbla-senkarzinom. *Therapiewoche* 1980; 30:6067.
36. Kowlakowski TS, Lamm DL: Intravesical therapy of superficial bladder cancer, in Resnick M (ed): *Current Trends in Urology,* vol 4. Baltimore, Williams & Wilkins Co, 1988, p 94.
37. Lamm DL, Crissman J, Blumenstein B, et al: Adriamycin versus BCG in su-perficial bladder cancer: A Southwest Oncology Group study, in Debruyne MJ, Denis L, van der Meijden APM (eds): *EORTC Genitourinary Group Monograph 6: BCG in Superficial Bladder Cancer.* New York, Alan R Liss Inc, 1989, p 263.
38. Lamm DL, Sarosdy MF, Grossman HB, et al: Maintenance vs. non-mainte-nance BCG immunotherapy of superficial bladder cancer: A Southwest Oncol-ogy Group study. Presented at the 85th annual meeting of the American Uro-logic Association, Dallas, Texas, May 1989.
39. Reynolds RH, Stogdill VD, Lamm DL: Disease progression in BCG treated pa-tients with transitional cell carcinoma of the bladder. *American Urologic Asso-ciation Proceedings* 1985; 133:390.
40. Lamm DL: BCG immunotherapy in bladder cancer. *J Urol* 1985; 134:40.
41. Debruyne FM: *Superficial Bladder Cancer Intravesical Therapy Trial: An In-terim Report.* Evansville, Bristol-Meyers, 1988.
42. Martinez-Pineiro JA, Leon JL, Martinez-Pineiro L Jr, et al: Bacillus Calmette-Guerin versus doxorubicin versus thiotepa: A randomized prospective study in 202 patients with superficial bladder cancer. *J Urol* 1990; 143:502.
43. Bretton PR, Herr HW, Kimmel M, et al: The response of patients with superfi-cial bladder cancer to a second course of intravesical bacillus Calmette-Guerin. *J Urol* 1990; 143:710.
44. Lamm DL, Sarosdy MF, DeHaven JI: Percutaneous, oral, or intravesical BCG administration: What is the optimal route?, in Debruyne MJ, Denis L, van der Meijden APM (eds): *EORTC Genitourinary Group Monograph 6: BCG in Su-perficial Bladder Cancer.* New York, Alan R Liss Inc, 1989, p 263.
45. Lamm DL, DeHaven JI, Shriver J, et al: A randomized prospective compari-son of oral versus intravesical and percutaneous bacillus Calmette-Guerin for superficial bladder cancer. *J Urol* 1990; 144:65.
46. Lamm DL, Steg A, Boccon-Gibod L, et al: Complications of bacillus Calmette-Guerin immunotherapy: Review of 2,602 patients and comparison of chemo-therapy complications, in Debruyne MJ, Denis L, van der Meijden APM (eds): *EORTC Genitourinary Group Monograph 6: BCG in Superficial Bladder Can-cer.* New York, Alan R Liss Inc, 1989, p 355.
47. Rawls WH, Lamm DL, Eyolfson MF: Septic complications in the use of bacil-lus Calmette-Guerin for non-invasive transitional cell carcinoma. *J Urol* 1988; 139:300.
48. Curtis JE, Hersh EM, Harris JE: The human primary immune response to key-hole limpet hemocyanin: Interrelationships of delayed hypersensitivity, anti-body response, and in vitro blast transformation. *Clin Exp Immunol* 1970; 6:473.
49. Olsson CA, Chute R, Rao CN: Immunologic reduction of bladder cancer rate. *J Urol* 1974; 111:173.
50. Jurincic CD, Engelmann U, Gasch J, et al: Immunotherapy in bladder cancer with keyhole limpet hemocyanin: Randomized study. 1988; *J Urol* 139:723.
51. Flamm OA, personal communication, Vienna, 1988.

Treatment of Invasive Bladder Cancer

James E. Montie, M.D.

Chairman, Department of Urology, Cleveland Clinic Florida, Fort Lauderdale, Florida

Bladder cancer is a heterogenous disease ranging from well-differentiated papillary lesions representing minimal threat to the patient to poorly differentiated tumors with a high potential for metastases even at the time of initial diagnosis. Although much effort has been extended to find better predictors of the risk posed by an individual bladder cancer, the histologic grade and tumor stage have remained the most important variables.[1] The ability of cancer cells to invade into the substance of the bladder wall identifies their lethal potential if incompletely treated. Although greater depth of invasion into the wall, increases the potential for spread, recent evidence emphasizes the significance of even lamina propria invasion as a harbinger of an aggressive cancer.[2, 3] Further penetration into the muscular wall increases the potential for metastatic spread in spite of successful local treatment, demonstrating the need for effective systemic treatment.

There are two fundamental issues facing the urologist in the management of bladder cancer: (1) when to remove the bladder because therapies cannot eliminate the local cancer, and (2) how to improve the survival of patients in whom there may be satisfactory control of the primary tumor but lethal metastases. The urologist's recommendation about the timing of bladder removal may be critical to the patient's survival.[4]

Recent data on effective chemotherapy for bladder cancer have raised expectations considerably.[5] The initial enthusiasm for cisplatin combinations has been tempered somewhat by the recognition of continuing relapse in patients achieving an initial complete response.[5, 6] The challenge now is the appropriate integration of chemotherapy with traditional treatment methods such as cystectomy or radiation therapy either (1) to improve patient survival, or (2) to preserve bladder function. The two goals must be separated clearly in order to allow proper judgments to be made. This review will examine two aspects of invasive bladder cancer that hold promise for improvements in survival, the selection of more appropriate therapy, or the reduction of morbidity.

Significance of T1 Disease

Since the classic staging system of Jewett and Strong was introduced in 1946, invasion of the lamina propria has been grouped with "superficial" tumors.[7] Although it was recognized that T1 (stage A) cancer was in fact "invasive," could be associated with metastases, and was more dangerous than Ta (stage O) cancer, its risk did not seem to warrant the extreme treatment available, i.e., cystectomy. Transurethral resection with or without intravesical chemotherapy was the usual approach, and it was only when the cancer invaded the muscular wall of the bladder that cystectomy was deemed necessary.

There is a better appreciation now of the risks of high-grade cancers. Grade III (poorly differentiated) noninvasive cancers *incompletely* treated are lethal, although the time to development of muscle invasion or metastases sometimes can be protracted. The risk of later muscle invasion with an initial T1 cancer is in the range of 50%.[2] Thus, the patient with a grade III, T1 cancer, with the urologist as his guide, must navigate the course of continued endoscopic management (preserving the bladder) vs. removal of the bladder with all the attendant negative effects of this operation. All urologists share a fear of continuing endoscopic management for too long and then performing cystectomy when it is too late.[4]

Discrimination between different types of T1 cancers is useful.[8] An isolated papillary lesion with lamina propria invasion can be removed by resecting the muscle beneath the cancer. If the tumor is resected entirely, further treatment, including removal of the bladder, will not accomplish any more. However, the situation often is not so simple. If other areas in the bladder harbor carcinoma in situ (CIS), resection only is unlikely to be effective. Intravesical agents, such as bacillus Calmette-Guerin, can be successful in this setting, as demonstrated by Herr.[9] If the cancer has been understaged or incompletely resected, it can recur in the bladder wall and intravesical treatment is unlikely to work. Definitive radiation therapy has been recommended and used successfully in Britain.[3]

Unsuspected lamina propria invasion can be seen when performing biopsies of areas of visually typical CIS. Since identification of the invasion in this manner is fortuitous, it is unknown if other areas in the bladder also harbor CIS with invasion. The effectiveness of topical intravesical treatment on disease invading the lamina propria is debatable.[3, 10] In this form of T1 disease, cystectomy may be appropriate, because identifying other areas of invasion may not be possible until gross disease is present.

A bladder cancer that penetrates the lamina propria demonstrates the biologic capacity of invasion, making it a potentially lethal disease. Failure to clear that patient's bladder may lead to his death. Although a brief trial (i.e., 6 months or less) of intravesical therapy may be valuable, delay of aggressive therapy until muscle invasion is evident is frequently ill-advised.[9]

Integrated Therapies for Local Control of Bladder Cancer

The 1980s produced a reevaluation of the quality of life issues associated with cystectomy and urinary diversion.[11, 12] The negative impact of a serious operation with 4 to 8 weeks of recovery, the permanent effect on urinary function imposed by all forms of diversion, and the usual disruption of sexual function cannot be denied or minimized. However, a consistent reduction in the risk and perioperative morbidity of cystectomy, the development of cutaneous and orthotopic continent urinary reservoirs, and the current feasibility of "nerve-sparing" cystectomy to preserve sexual function testify to the progress made in ameliorating the consequences of this procedure, which presently is the most effective treatment available.[13-15] The introduction of chemotherapy regimens with the ability to induce complete remission of metastatic transitional cell carcinoma produced interest in their use in localized disease in an effort to achieve bladder preservation.[16] Radiation therapy alone is used widely in Canada and Great Britain in place of cystectomy.[3] Chemotherapy combined with radiation therapy could improve results further. Data to evaluate these "bladder preservation" protocols are preliminary and intriguing.

The bladder preservation approach is contrasted with a "bladder reconstruction" philosophy in which new methods of urinary diversion with continent cutaneous or orthotopic reservoirs are used to restore the functional aspects of a "bladder" and to improve life-style. With this approach, systemic chemotherapy can be integrated with cystectomy, either before or after operation, to improve survival by treating micrometastases. This review will examine the advantages and limitations of each of these approaches (Tables 1 and 2).

Bladder Preservation

Sternberg and associates at Memorial Sloan-Kettering Cancer Center (MSKCC) reported in 1985 the initial results with the M-VAC regimen (methotrexate, vinblastine [Velban], doxorubicin [Adriamycin] and cisplatin).[17] Similar response rates were reported with the CMV protocol (cisplatin, methotrexate, and vinblastine [Velban]).[18, 19] The recent review of the MSKCC experience provides the most complete data available to date.[6]

Most response rates were based on experience with metastatic disease. However, in patients with bladder in place, response rates in the pelvis have been comparable or better than those seen at other soft tissue sites.[6, 18, 19] The complete response rate in the MSKCC series was 36% ± 9%, with an overall response (partial or complete response) rate of 72% ± 8%.[6] In patients with lymph node involvement, the complete response rate was higher (52%). These data support the concept of bladder preservation. However, several key points that impact on the use of chemotherapy deserve emphasis. First, 68% of the patients achieving a complete re-

TABLE 1.
Bladder Preservation

For	Against

Chemotherapy (M-VAC)
  Partial response: 60% to 70%
  Complete response: 20% to 30%
  (stage-dependent)
	Presumably not beneficial to
	  nonresponders

Maintains good sexual and bladder
  function
	Delays cystectomy in 50% to 80% not
	  achieving complete response

May be feasible in patients not
  suitable for cystectomy
	Restaging error is 30% to 40% (cTo
	  but P+)

Primary tumor may allow evaluation
  of response
	Chemotherapy and radiation therapy
	  work poorly against mucosal disease

Chemotherapy tolerated better than
  postoperatively
	Chemotherapy and radiation therapy
	  work poorly against nontransitional
	  elements (i.e., squamous cell and
	  adenocarcinoma)

Theoretic benefit of early treatment of
  micrometastases
	New tumors not prevented and
	  follow-up cystoscopy needed

Partial cystectomy may be feasible in
  selected patients
	Morbidity and mortality of
	  chemotherapy with or without
	  radiation therapy

Combined chemotherapy and
  radiation may raise complete
  response rate to 50% to 80%
	Possible later increased morbidity of
	  cystectomy

	Longer length of treatment compared to cystectomy alone

	Possible cumulative toxicity on
	  bladder function if intravesical
	  treatment is needed

sponse later relapsed. In addition, the toxicity with M-VAC was substantial. There was a 25% rate of nadir-sepsis, a 49% rate of mucositis (13% severe), and a 3% rate of drug-related mortality. Toxicity in patients without metastases may be less because of a better pretherapy performance status. The CMV regimen has a response comparable to that of the M-VAC.[18, 19] The complete response in the bladder is 25% ± 11% with a partial response rate of 16% ± 9%.[20] Some concern persists about the amount of improvement afforded by M-VAC or CMV compared to cisplatin alone, and prospective trials are needed to address this specific question.[21]

The data evaluating systemic chemotherapy for locally advanced but resectable disease (T2-T4NXM0) are limited. Although the primary tumor responds in a manner similar to those in other soft tissue sites, issues such as the influence of mucosal disease (carcinoma in situ), restaging errors, and

TABLE 2.
Bladder Reconstruction

Quickest elimination of local cancer	Loss of normal bladder function
Lowest pelvic/bladder recurrence rate	Frequent loss of potency in men
Precise determination of pathologic stage	Operative mortality 1% to 3%
Can be combined with adjuvant or neoadjuvant chemotherapy	Reoperation rate 10% to 30%
Eliminates development of new bladder cancers and need for cystoscopy	Undefined late consequences of urinary reservoirs (metabolic abnormalities, anemia, bowel cancers, etc.)

the development of new tumors are important.[6, 18, 19] Herr has described the MSKCC experience of initial chemotherapy in 50 patients with T2-4N0M0 disease who received a median of two cycles of M-VAC.[22] Forty-four patients were evaluable for clinical response; 55% (24 of 44) were stage T0 posttreatment by Transurethral resection biopsies (TUR-BT). Noteworthy is the observation that the addition of computed tomographic scans decreased the complete response rate to 22% (12 of 44). Of these 12 patients, 8 were indeed pathologic complete response. Twenty of the 50 patients refused postchemotherapy surgery because of an apparent favorable response, relief of symptoms, and the desire to preserve bladder function. Only 6 of 20 patients (30%) remain free of cancer with an intact bladder, and 5 have recurrent or new superficial disease being managed with intravesical treatment. Thirty patients had no residual disease, suggesting that bladder preservation may be possible for them. Overall, it appears that 25% to 40% of patients can be rendered free of cancer in their bladder with chemotherapy, but as many as half of these will develop local recurrence later. Thus, long-term control in the pelvis without cystectomy may be only in the range of 15% to 25%. More chemotherapy (i.e., four cycles vs. two cycles) and the selection of patients with a smaller tumor burden (complete response rates of 100% for stage T2, 56% for stage T3, and 42% for stage T4) may improve these results.

The Cleveland Clinic has experience with a phase I–II trial of M-VAC in which the cisplatin is delivered intra-arterially.[23] Although technically feasible and adequately tolerated at a dose of 100 mg/m^2 of cisplatin, the therapeutic advantage of this route of administration over intravenous therapy is only speculative.

A logical extension is the combination of chemotherapy and radiation therapy to preserve the bladder. Early experience was with cisplatin alone (100 mg/m^2 × 3 weeks) followed by definitive radiation therapy. Thirty-eight of 50 patients (76%) were said to have been managed without the need for cystectomy.[24] A National Bladder Cancer Collaborative Group Trial of cisplatin and radiation therapy yielded 36 of 70 patients (51%) maintaining the bladder without recurrence.[25] The University of Florida study has used two cycles of CMV or M-VAC followed by concurrent definitive radiation therapy (6,480 rads total tumor dose) and low-dose cisplatin (10 mg/m^2/wk × 7).[16] Twelve of 30 (44%) patients completing the initial chemotherapy had a complete response. A trial in Germany of cisplatin (25 mg/m^2/day × 5 days on first and fifth week) combined with moderate-dose radiation therapy (50 Gy) led to resolution of the cancer and normal bladder function in 83% of patients.[26] The combination of intraarterial cisplatin and concurrent radiation therapy has been explored by Eapen and associates, who identified a clinical complete response rate of 23 out of 25 patients (92%).[27]

The experience of Shipley et al. has been evaluated thoroughly.[28] The regimen includes initial CMV × 2 and then a combination of radiation therapy and cisplatin in patients who have a favorable response, the goal being bladder preservation with early cystectomy reserved for those who do not respond. Forty-four patients entered the protocol; 43% (19 of 44) have completed the study and maintained bladder function without a recurrence. The prospects for continuing progress in efforts at bladder preservation are intriguing and need to be pursued. The initial experience indicates several important points:

1. Patients who respond do so quickly, within one or two cycles. Failure to obtain a complete response with either chemotherapy alone or radiation therapy combined with chemotherapy indicates the need for a cystectomy.

2. Patients unable to tolerate full-dose chemotherapy may not be appropriate candidates for initial treatment because no data are available regarding the efficacy of substantially reduced doses.[21]

3. Mucosal disease (CIS) responds less well to systemic chemotherapy, radiation therapy, or combination treatments.

4. When squamous cell or adenocarcinomatous elements are present with transitional cell carcinoma, the response is poor.[6] Frequently, the nontransitional elements persist after elimination of the transitional cells.

5. The restaging error after chemotherapy is in the range of 30% to 50% and after combined radiation therapy and chemotherapy may be higher.[6, 22]

6. Chemotherapy or radiation therapy does not prevent the development of new cancers in the bladder; thus, continuing endoscopic surveillance is necessary.[6, 28]

7. The cumulative toxicity of integrated therapy must be considered. Two or three cycles of systemic chemotherapy followed by radiation therapy takes approximately 4 to 6 months. The addition of intravesical treatment, such as bacillus Calmette-Guerin, may adversely affect bladder function. The potential increased risk of a salvage cystectomy after failure of all of the above treatments is not defined.

Bladder Reconstruction

Concurrent with the availability of more effective chemotherapy, progress in surgery for bladder cancer also has been made in three areas:

1. Use of methods for continent urinary diversion.
2. Lower operative mortality.
3. Potential for "nerve-sparing" cystoprostatectomy.

Interest in urinary diversions as an alternative to the ileal conduit resurfaced approximately 10 years ago with the studies of Kock et al.[29] The motivation for this was not based on failure of the ileal conduit as a safe and reliable diversion in the adult cancer patient, but on a desire to improve the patient's quality of life by avoiding the need for an external appliance. The continent ileal reservoir was improved and popularized by Skinner and associates.[30] Initial reoperation rates, due almost exclusively to efferent valve malfunction, were in the range of 20% to 30%; these have decreased notably to 10% to 15% with modifications in surgical technique. The complexity in construction of the ileal reservoir stimulated the use of other bowel segments, mostly right colonic and ileocolonic segments, with a number of modifications in the methods used for achieving continence. The relative superiority of ileal or right hemicolonic reservoirs is not germane to this review, but it is clear that in some patients a continent cutaneous reservoir without the need for a collecting device is an attractive alternative that leads to better rehabilitation.

Probably the best bladder reconstruction allows voiding through the urethra.[13, 14] Although earlier operations such as the Camey procedure (tubular ileal reservoir) were associated with disappointingly high rates of both daytime and nighttime incontinence, newer reservoirs that have a large volume, a low pressure, and a high compliance provide for very good daytime continence (85%) and good nocturnal continence (50% to 90%). The urethral reservoir should be offered to all male patients with the following constraints: there should be relatively low risk for urethral recurrence, good general health, and tolerance of the potential for nocturnal enuresis. This operation eliminates the stoma, preserves body image, and probably lessens the risk of bacteriuria.

An augmented rectal reservoir is a modification of a ureterosigmoidostomy and can be particularly valuable to the male who has a high risk for urethral disease or the female who wishes to avoid a urinary stoma.[30] The largest contemporary experience comes from Egypt and affirms acceptable results in their patient population. Passing a combination of urine and feces may be a significant problem for some patients, but the results with the improved techniques should be better than those seen with the classical ureterosigmoidostomy.

Cystectomy historically has been the most dangerous operation performed by a urologist. Improved perioperative care including volume status monitoring, nutritional evaluation and support, bowel preparation by mechanical cleansing and antibacterials, intraoperative anesthesia monitoring, and blood product replacement has allowed the operation to be performed with a lower morbidity and mortality. Mortality rates ranging from 0.4% to 2.5% have been reported recently and a goal of 1% to 2% should be attainable.[13] The surgery is still very demanding for the patient and recovery takes 4 to 8 weeks.

Modifications in the technique of radical prostatectomy to spare the nerves controlling erectile function also can be applied to a cystoprostatectomy, thereby preserving potency.[15] The dissection needs to be closer to the bladder, seminal vesicles, and bladder neck than is done in the classical technique, but in selected patients this approach should not raise the risk for pelvic recurrences appreciably.[31] Thus, for the male patient, we have the ability to provide a very functional voiding pattern with low operative risk and the possible maintenance of erectile function.

Perspective

In evaluating integrated therapies for high-stage bladder cancer, the goal of the treatment must be kept foremost. Systemic chemotherapy may improve survival without allowing more bladders to be preserved; on the other hand, while it may allow more bladders to be preserved, it may not improve or may even decrease overall survival. Bladder preservation and improved survival are both admirable goals; to evaluate the impact of chemotherapy effectively, we must maintain these goals and design the appropriate studies.

The research of investigators such as Shipley et al. and Wajsman et al. is aimed at bladder preservation (possibly with the additional benefit of improved survival).[16, 28] Quality of life issues, morbidity of treatments, and late local results are key end points. Careful point selection likely will be important to optimize the bladder preservation approach.

An Intergroup Study now in progress examines three courses of systemic M-VAC neoadjuvant chemotherapy vs. cystectomy alone and is designed to evaluate the impact of these treatments on survival. It does not address the issue of bladder preservation. This study is extremely important and should add significantly to our knowledge about the value of chemotherapy for high-stage bladder cancer. If it is found that chemotherapy improves the survival rate over cystectomy alone, the best use of chemotherapy will need to be determined (i.e., neoadjuvant treatment or classical adjuvant therapy). Skinner et al. now have data indicating that cisplatin, doxorubicin, and cyclophosphamide after cystectomy and pelvic node dissection improve both time to progression and survival.[32]

Therapy for high-stage bladder cancer is improving, both in terms of substitute procedures, rehabilitation after cystectomy, and bladder preservation. Our challenge is to avoid the single-minded attitude that presumes that one approach is best for all patients.

References

1. Whitmore WF Jr: Bladder cancer: An overview. *CA* 1988; 38:213–223.
2. Jakse G, Loidl W, Seeber G, et al: Stage T1, grade 3 transitional cell carcinoma of the bladder: An unfavorable tumor. *J Urol* 1987; 137:39–43.
3. Jenkins B, Nauth-Misir R, Martin JE, et al: The fate of G3pT1 bladder cancer. *Br J Urol* 1989; 64:608–610.
4. Wood DP Jr, Montie JE: Bladder cancer: Deciding on appropriate surgery. *Oncology* 1989; 3:55–61.
5. Sternberg CN, Scher HI: Current status on chemotherapy for urothelial tract tumors. *Oncology* 1987; 1:41–48.
6. Sternberg CN, Yagoda A, Scher H, et al: Methotrexate, vinblastine, doxorubicin, and cisplatin for advanced transitional cell carcinoma of the urethelium. *Cancer* 1989; 64:2448–2458.
7. Jewett HJ, Strong GH: Infiltrating carcinoma of the bladder: Relation of depth of penetration of the bladder wall to incidence of local extension and metastases. *J Urol* 1946; 55:366–372.
8. Masters JRW, Camplejohn RS, Parkinson MC, et al: DNA ploidy and the prognosis of stage pT1 bladder cancer. *Br J Urol* 1989; 64:403–408.
9. Herr HW, Badalament RA, Amato DA, et al: Superficial bladder cancer treated with bacillus calmette-guerin: A multivariate analysis of factors affecting tumor progression. *J Urol* 1989; 141:22–29.
10. Droller MJ, Walsh PC: Intensive intravesical chemotherapy in the treatment of flat carcinoma in situ: Is it safe? *J Urol* 1985; 134:1115–1117.
11. Montie JE, Pontes JE, Smyth EM: Selection of the type of urinary diversion in conjunction with radical cystectomy. *J Urol* 1987; 137:1154–1155.
12. Mansson ASA, Johnson G, Mansson W: Quality of life after cystectomy: Comparison between patients with conduit and those with continent caecal reservoir urinary diversion. *Br J Urol* 1988; 62:240–254.
13. Montie JE, Wood DP Jr: The risk of radical cystectomy. *Br J Urol* 1988; 63:483–486.
14. Skinner DG, Lieskovsky G, Boyd S: Continent urinary diversion. *J Urol* 1989; 141:1323–1327.
15. Schlegel PN, Walsh P: Neuroanatomical approach to radical cystoprostatectomy with preservation of sexual function. *J Urol* 1987; 138:1402–1406.
16. Wajsman Z, Klimberg IW: Treatment alternatives for invasive bladder cancer. *Semin Surg Oncol* 1989; 5:72–81.
17. Steinberg CN, Yagoda A, Scher HI, et al: Preliminary results of MVAC (methotrexate, vinblastine, doxorubicin and cisplatin) for transitional cell carcinoma of the urothelium. *J Urol* 1985; 133:403–407.
18. Meyers FJ, Palmer JM, Freiha FS, et al: The fate of the bladder in patients with metastatic bladder cancer treated with cisplatin, methotrexate and vinblastine: A Northern California Oncology Group Study. *J Urol* 1985; 134:1118–1121.
19. Wahle SM, Williams RD, Gerstbrein JJ, et al: CMV chemotherapy for extensive urothelial carcinoma. *World J Urol* 1988; 6:158–162.
20. Myers FJ, Palmer JM, Hannigan JF: Chemotherapy of disseminated transitional cell carcinoma, in William RD (ed): *Advances in Urologic Oncology. volume 1, General Perspectives.* New York, Macmillan, 1988, pp 83–192.
21. Scher HI: Should single agents be standard therapy for urothelial tract tumors? *J Clin Oncol* 1989; 7:694–697.

22. Herr HW: Neoadjuvant chemotherapy for invasive bladder cancer. *Semin Surg Oncol* 1989; 5:266–271.
23. Montie JE, Bukowski RM, Pontes JE, et al: Intra-arterial chemotherapy for localized carcinoma of the bladder, in Johnson DE, Logothetis CJ, Von Eschenbach AC (eds): *Systemic Therapy for Genitourinary Cancers.* Chicago, Year Book Medical Publishers, 1989, pp 64–72.
24. Raghavan D, Pearson B, Duval P, et al: Initial intravenous cis-platinum therapy: Improved management for invasive high risk bladder cancer? *J Urol* 1985; 133:399–402.
25. Shipley WU, Prout GR Jr, Einstein AB, et al: Treatment of invasive bladder cancer by cisplatin and radiation in patients unsuited for surgery. *JAMA* 1987; 258:931–935.
26. Sauer MD, Schrott KM, Dunst J, et al: Preliminary results of treatment of invasive bladder carcinoma with radiotherapy and cisplatin. *J Radiat Oncol* 1988; 15:871–875.
27. Eapen L, Stewart D, Danjoux C, et al: Intraarterial cisplatin and concurrent radiation for locally advanced bladder cancer. *J Clin Oncol* 1989; 7:230–235.
28. Shipley WU, Prout GR, Kaufman DS: Bladder cancer: Advances in laboratory innovations and clinical management, with emphasis or innovations allowing bladder-sparing approaches for patients with invasive tumors. *Cancer* 1990; 65:675–683.
29. Kock NG, Norlen L, Philipson BM, et al: The continent ileal reservoir (Kock pouch) for urinary diversion. *World J Urol* 1985; 3:146–151.
30. Kock NG, Ghoneim MA, Lycke KG, et al: Urinary diversion to the augmented and valved rectum: Preliminary results with a novel surgical procedure. *J Urol* 1988; 140:1375–1379.
31. Pritchett TR, Schiff WM, Klatt E, et al: The potency-sparing radical cystectomy: Does it compromise the completeness of the cancer resection? *J Urol* 1988; 140:1400–1403.
32. Skinner DG, Daniels JR, Reissel CA, et al: The role of adjuvant chemotherapy following cystectomy for invasive bladder cancer: A prospective study. *J Urol* 1990; 143:290.

Endocrine Management of Prostate Cancer

Fritz H. Schröder, M.D.

Professor and Chairman, Department of Urology, Erasmus University, Rotterdam, The Netherlands

Claus G. Röhrborn, M.D.

Division of Urology, Southwestern Medical School, University of Texas Southwestern Medical Center at Dallas, Dallas, Texas

Hormones and Prostate Cancer

In animals as well as in humans, the prostate depends on androgens in its development, growth, and function. Related evidence has been reviewed by Coffey and Isaacs in 1981.[1] Similarly, prostate cancer in men seems to be androgen-dependent in its development and, in many instances, after it has progressed to clinically relevant disease. There is anecdotal evidence that prostate cancer does not occur in early castrates.[2] This scanty evidence seems to show that androgens play at least a permissive role in the pathogenesis of this disease. In the morphogenesis of human prostate cancer, several steps can be identified. Focal disease, usually well-differentiated prostate cancer found at autopsy, is 800 to 1,000 times more frequent than clinical prostate cancer in the western world. As described by Yatani and coworkers[3] at the same time, the incidence of clinical disease in some regions of the world, such as China and Japan, may be more than ten times lower than in western countries. Because of the increase in incidence observed in migrants from Japan to Hawaii and the U.S. mainland, described by Akazaki and coworkers,[4] environmental factors have been investigated by epidemiologists to explain the different rate of promotion from focal to clinical disease in various areas of the world. Observations made by Hämäläinen et al.[5] show that a vegetarian diet may lead to a significant decrease in plasma testosterone and other related hormones. de Jong et al.[6] found significantly lower levels of plasma testosterone in Japanese as compared to Dutch males. On the basis of such observations, the possibility that regional differences in the incidence of clinical prostate cancer may be explained by variations in the endocrine environment cannot be excluded. Plasma testosterone seems to have at least a permissive, and possibly a promoting, function in the pathogenesis of the disease.

Normal prostatic development depends on an androgenic stimulus afforded predominantly by testicular testosterone.[7] In the adult male, total plasma testosterone amounts to 5.72 ± 1.35 µg/L (18.9 ± 4.7 nmol/L), and in the adult female it amounts to 0.37 ± 0.10 µg/L (1.3 ± 0.3 nmol/L). Testosterone is produced by the Leydig cells in the testes under the control of luteinizing hormone and the hypothalamic pituitary axis. Various feedback mechanisms involved in its regulation are schematically indicated in Figure 1.

Adrenal androgens, androstenedione and dihydroepiandrosterone are produced in the zonae fasciculata and reticularis of the adrenal cortex under the control of adrenocorticotropic hormone (ACTH) released from the anterior pituitary gland. ACTH release is stimulated by corticotropic releasing factor from the hypothalamus. Adrenal androgens do not mediate negative feedback on ACTH secretion, for which cortisol is the most important feedback signal. Adrenal androgens are weak compared to testosterone or dihydrotestosterone (DHT) and are bound almost completely to albumin.

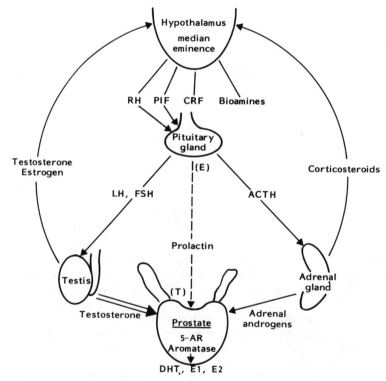

FIG 1.
Endocrine factors regulating prostatic growth and function. *RH* = releasing hormones; *PIF* = pituitary factor for prolactin; *E* = estrogen; *LH* = luteinizing hormone; *FSH* = follicle-stimulating hormone; *ACTH* = adrenocorticotropic hormone; *T* = testosterone; *DHT* = 5α-dihydrotestosterone; *5-AR* = 5α-reductase; *CRF* = corticotropin releasing factor.

Adrenal androgens may be metabolized to testosterone and dihydrotestosterone. They account for the plasma testosterone levels measured after castration that amount to roughly one-tenth of the original values.

The balance of production, metabolism, and plasma binding determines the amount of biologically active testosterone available in the target cells. Inside the prostate cell, testosterone is converted to DHT by the enzyme 5-α-reductase. Both testosterone and DHT, the latter with higher affinity, bind within the target cell to specific androgen receptors. Ligand binding appears to activate the receptor, which results in modulation of gene transcription, the exact mechanisms of which are just beginning to be understood. The recent cloning and characterization of the human androgen receptor (by Tilley[8] and three other groups) has provided researchers with an important and powerful tool with which to start unraveling some of these questions.

Endocrine treatment is usually applied to patients with advanced metastatic disease, which is diagnosed in more than half of all clinical cases. Consequently, the majority of patients present initially with systemic disease and require some form of systemic treatment. Such a systemic form of treatment was introduced in 1941 by Huggins et al.,[9] who demonstrated that prostate cancer is androgen-dependent like normal prostatic epithelium. In the following decades it was established that a reduction of serum testosterone to castrate levels would result in a 70% initial subjective response rate in symptomatic patients with metastatic prostate cancer. However, it also was found that the initial response rate was followed by a relapse after 1 to 3 years of hormonal deprivation treatment, despite continued low testosterone levels. This relapse also is called the "escape" phenomenon and is thought to be due to the growth of cells that are either primarily hormone-unresponsive or have become hormone-independent.[10] Therefore, hormonal deprivation therapy for metastatic prostatic carcinoma must be considered as a form of systemic palliative treatment. Also, many patients with prostate cancer die *with* their disease rather than *of* their disease; cure by means of endocrine management, in the sense of complete disappearance of all prostate cancer, rarely has been described.

Some of the essential questions of endocrine management of prostate cancer are still open. It is not known whether endocrine treatment will prolong life, whether early or delayed treatment is preferable, or whether patients with localized disease would benefit from endocrine treatment. There is also uncertainty about the best method of hormonal deprivation treatment. Adrenal androgens are insufficient to promote normal prostatic development and to maintain normal function of the prostatic epithelium, as has been shown by Oesterling et al.[11] However, cancer may behave differently and, at present, major efforts are undertaken to rule out or confirm the possibility that the exclusion of adrenal androgens together with testicular androgens may be associated with an improvement of survival in metastatic prostate cancer. Prior to dealing with the various methods of endocrine treatment and the results obtained, some important aspects of endocrine dependence of human prostate cancer will be reviewed.

Endocrine Dependence of Human Prostate Cancer

Human prostatic carcinoma either becomes hormone-independent during the natural course of its development, or hormone-resistant populations of cells are present even in very small tumors from their inception. Evidence resulting from animal models on this subject has been reviewed by Isaacs and Kyprianou.[12] The variability in response observed between different patients affected by the disease under endocrine treatment may be explained by competition of clonal growth of different cell populations. Different types of endocrine management also may be associated with different response rates.

Response to Endocrine Treatment

Response rates reported in the literature are extremely variable. This is due mainly to the different sets of response criteria used in various studies. Frequently used are the response criteria of the National Prostatic Cancer Project (NPCP) as described by Murphy and Slack,[13] and those of the European Organization for Research on Treatment of Cancer (EORTC), as described by Schröder[14] and Newling.[15] The major difference between these two sets of criteria lies in the fact that the NPCP recommends the use of stable disease as a classification of objective response. Unfortunately, as long as no reproducibly measurable parameters are found that correlate with the prognosis of the individual patient, uncertainty in judging response and progression will remain. Measurable lesions are rare in prostatic cancer.

The early studies of the EORTC genitourinary group were among the first that established response rates by strictly defined criteria. Complete and partial remission rates found in protocols 30761 and 30762 are reproduced in Table 1.[16, 17] Irrespective of the differences between the two studies in which the same response criteria were used, and irrespective of a significant difference that was found in protocol 30761 in the disadvantage of medroxyprogesterone acetate, it is evident that response rates are rather low if stabilization is excluded. Stable disease in most studies using the NPCP criteria amounts to 40% to 50% if included in an estimation of best response. It is also evident that response and progression rates are different for primary tumors and metastases. In the two EORTC studies, these differences are statistically significant. Rectal examination was used to judge local response and progression.

If rectal examination is replaced by volume measurements with transrectal ultrasonography, which has been found to be reproducible within 5% to 10%, the same findings are obtained. Carpentier et al. found a volume reduction of the prostate in virtually all previously untreated patients averaging 40% after 3 months of treatment.[18, 19] Within a 1-year period, distant progression occurred in 20 of 55 patients, while a noticeable increase

TABLE 1.
Best Response Rates to Endocrine Treatment in Protocols 30761 and 30762 of the EORTC Genitourinary Group*

Protocol	Agent†	Local N	Local %	Distant N	Distant %	Progression N	Progression %
30761	CPA	24	(40)	5	(13)	39	(52)
	MPA	15	(26)	1	(3)	48	(68)
	DES	31	(55)	5	(18)	30	(47)
30762	DES	51	(51.5)	16	(31.4)	–	–
	EMP	35	(35.0)	11	(24.4)	–	–

*Data from Pavone-Macaluso M, de Vogt HJ, Viggiano G, et al: *J Urol* 1986; 136:624–631 and Smith PH, Suciu S, Robinson MRG, et al: *J Urol* 1986; 136:619–623.
†DES = diethylstilbestrol; EMP = estramustine phosphate; CPA = cyproterone acetate; MPA = medroxyprogesterone acetate.

of the primary tumor was seen in only 2 patients. Sneller[20] showed that the initial decrease in primary tumor volume correlates with the prognosis and rate of progression. Multivariate analysis, however, failed to demonstrate superiority of this parameter as a prognostic indicator if compared to grade and stage. These findings are very suggestive for the presence of different cell populations with respect to hormone responsiveness in primary tumors and metastases of human prostate cancer.

Endocrine Dependence and Cell Death

In the few available animal models of prostate cancer (in hormone-dependent transplantable human tumor lines in nude mice) and in measurable lesions in humans, response to endocrine treatment is indicated by a decrease of tumor mass. Evidence is accumulating that cell death due to androgen withdrawal is not just a passive phenomenon leading to tumor cell necrosis. Using the ventral prostate of the rat as a model, Isaacs[21] has shown that different concentrations of androgen are associated with different rates of cell death. Montpetit and coworkers[22] have produced evidence that cell death is an active cellular process. Proteins that otherwise are not detected in prostate cells appear after androgen withdrawal, leading to cell death. Humphries and Isaacs,[23] using the Dunning R3327-3 rat prostatic adenocarcinoma cell line, showed that cell loss is associated with high intracellular testosterone concentrations but low DHT. A better understanding of the mechanisms involved in cell death may allow more selective and efficient manipulation of this process.

Minimal Amounts of Androgens and Growth Response

It must be assumed that the concentration of androgens found in the tissue of the normal human prostate, benign prostatic hyperplasia, or prostatic cancer are capable of exerting the functional and growth effects that are characteristic for these different prostatic tissues. Some of the data obtained from the literature are summarized in Table 2. Some of the differences seen are due to methodological difficulties and the handling of tissue prior to the study. Walsh and coworkers[29] have pointed out that it is of crucial importance whether fresh prostatic tissue or that obtained by autopsy is studied. Both benign prostatic hyperplasia and prostatic cancer tissues in the intact male contain more DHT than testosterone.

As we mentioned before, plasma testosterone after castration will decrease to about 10% of its original level. Androgen levels in human prostate cancer tissue after castration were first reported by Geller and coworkers.[26] They found that, on the average, DHT levels in castrated males drop to 30% to 40% of those found in intact males. In a series of 20 castrated patients who relapsed after initial response to treatment, all but 2 prostatic cancer tissues showed levels below 2.4 ng/g of tissue, which is equivalent to about 9 pmol/g. The critical question regarding whether the amount of androgen remaining after castration is still capable of stimulating prostatic cancer tissue to grow cannot be answered at this moment. Labrie et al.[31] found in studying the androgen-dependent SC-115 Shionogi mammary carcinoma cell line a wide variation of androgen sensitivity in clones of cells derived from single cell plating. Although the remaining androgen production after castration in humans is not capable of maintaining prostatic growth and function, the possibility cannot be excluded that cancer cells

TABLE 2.
Endogenous Testosterone and Dihydrotestosterone Concentrations in Normal Phosphate, Benign Prostatic Hyperplasia and Prostate Cancer in pmol/g of Tissue

Study	Normal Prostate		Benign Prostatic Hyperplasia		Prostate Cancer	
	T*	DHT	T	DHT	T	DHT
Habib[24]	–	–	14	45	40	22
Ghanadian[25]	–	–	1.3	25	7.0	12
Geller[26]	–	7.0	–	18	–	10
Krieg[27]	0.8	6.0	1.1	17	4.5	15
Siiteri[28]	4.0	4.5	4.0	20	–	–
Walsh[29]	4.0	18	6.0	18	–	–
Bolton[30]	–	–	0.9	18	–	–

*T = testosterone; DHT = dihydrotestosterone.

may be more sensitive to androgenic stimuli than normal prostatic epithelial cells.

The androgen-dependent humanprostatic carcinoma cell line PC-82 has been used to study the effect of various concentrations of androgens on proliferation markers and growth in nude mice. There was cessation of growth with plasma testosterone levels in the range of 0.8 nmol/L, which corresponded to DHT concentrations in the tumor of 3 to 4 pmol/g of tissue. Lower DHT levels led to further volume decrease.[32] In other experiments by van Steenbrugge,[33] the minimal DHT concentration in tumor tissue that would stimulate proliferation was in the range of 12 to 14 pmol/g of tissue. On the basis of these findings, the possibility cannot be excluded that relatively high concentrations of DHT in the tumor following castration could lead in some patients to a stimulation of growth. These and other findings have been used as an argument for total androgen ablation, including adrenal androgens, in the primary management of metastatic prostate cancer by Labrie and coworkers.[34]

Which Androgens Stimulate Prostate Cancer to Grow?

At this time, it is uncertain whether cancer of the prostate is stimulated preferentially by DHT (in analogy to the developing human prostate), as has been claimed by some investigators.[35] Since the enzyme 5α-reductase, which converts testosterone to DHT, can be blocked by potent and clinically available inhibitors, this mechanism could be exploited if indeed prostate cancer is more dependent on DHT than on testosterone. Such a regimen would have the additional advantage of maintaining potency and libido, both of which are dependent mainly on testosterone. The exploitation of this mechanism, however, is purely hypothetical at the moment. Other mechanisms that may be involved in prostatic growth will be dealt with when discussing the various methods of endocrine treatment for prostate cancer.

Methods of Endocrine Treatment and Treatment Results

Orchiectomy

Orchiectomy is the gold standard in hormonal deprivation therapy of prostate cancer against which all other treatment modalities have to be compared. In their original report, Huggins et al.[36] demonstrated that 15 of 21 (71%) patients with metastatic prostate cancer had subjective improvement in pain and/or objective improvement in neurological symptoms after bilateral orchiectomy. They also noted a decrease in the serum acid phosphatase as a response to hormonal deprivation in those patients who did respond favorably, a parameter for hormone-responsiveness that is still in use today. Bilateral orchiectomy reduces circulating testosterone levels from 20 μmol/L to 2 μmol/L, the so-called castrate level, in a very short period of time. Equally important is the fact that the testosterone level will remain in the castrate range for the remainder of the patient's life, as described by Robinson.[37] It is thought that in this way growth of the androgen-dependent population of cells is permanently arrested. In 1942, Riba[38] introduced a modification of the surgical technique, the subcapsular orchiectomy. With this technique, the tunica albuginea and the epididymis remain in situ offering a more acceptable cosmetic result. The debate over whether subcapsular orchiectomy is as effective as total orchiectomy has been put to the test by several recent studies, which showed that testosterone levels are indeed lowered to castrate levels by the modified procedure, and remain low even after human chorionic gonadotropin stimulation.[39, 40]

Bilateral orchiectomy offers several advantages over all other forms of androgen ablation: it is a minor operation that can be performed under local anesthesia; it can be performed on almost any patient in any clinical condition; the therapeutic response is almost immediate; there is no need for prolonged medication and no risk of drug-related side effects; and there is no concern about patient compliance. The disadvantages of the associated psychological trauma, may be decreased by the cosmetically more pleasing subcapsular orchiectomy. Unfortunately, the almost certain loss of libido and potency is common to most forms of androgen deprivation.

Bilateral Adrenalectomy

The ablation of adrenal androgens has been used in the past as a second-line endocrine treatment. Its use in the context of total androgen blockade as initial treatment together with orchiectomy or other modalities to remove or counteract testicular androgens will be discussed later. Persistent androgen production by the adrenal cortex has long been perceived as a possible basis for ultimate relapse after primary hormonal deprivation. Consequently, surgical and medical adrenalectomy as well as hypophysectomy have been proposed, and many reports have been published claiming some form of response to these forms of therapy in patients who relapsed after orchiectomy or primary estrogen treatment. Most of the results of phase II studies available from the literature are summarized in Table 3. With the use of very variable response criteria, an average of 34% of objective responses with a mean duration of 2.5 months was seen in 116 patients. Subjective response, mainly pain relief, was seen in 74% of patients and lasted an average of 4 months. The results obtained by these authors are not comparable because of variation in patient selection and response criteria. Considering the expected strong placebo effect, the reported subjective response rates probably represent an overestimation of the effectiveness of adrenalectomy. In view of the short duration of response and the need for glucocorticoid replacement after bilateral adrenalectomy, it is not surprising that this form of treatment did not find widespread acceptance. However, there seems to be some effect of secondary withdrawal of adrenal androgens in patients who progress after orchiectomy.

TABLE 3.
Results of Bilateral Adrenalectomy as a Second-Line Endocrine Treatment of Metastatic Prostatic Carcinoma

Author	Number of Patients	Objective Response		Subjective Response	
		Proportion	Duration	Proportion	Duration
Huggins[41]	4	—		1/4	Unknown
West[42]	10	1/10	3 mos	7/10	14–220, Average 83 days
Harrison[43]	7	3/7	Unknown	5/10 Pain 6/10 Activity	Unknown Unknown
Baker[44]	10	0	—	8/10 Pain 7/10 Activity	3 wks–6 mos
Scardino[45]	3	1/3 Local 3/3 AP*	2–4 mos	3/3 Pain and activity	3–9 mos
Taylor[46]	6	2/6 Mass 2/6 AP*	247–387 days	5/6 Pain	90–150 days
Morales[47]	20	1/18 Local	Unknown	9/10 Pain 4/10 Complete 5/10 Partial	Unknown
MacFarlane[48]	13	Unknown		9/13 Pain activity, weight	2–46 mos
Schoonees[49]	13	11/13 AP*	1.05 ± 0.33	11/13 Pain	1.98 ± 0.23 mos
Mahony[50]	22	8/22 Mass, cancer, and AP*	Unknown	18/22 Pain	Unknown
Totals	116	34% (27/79)	2.5 mos	74% (75/101)	4.0 mos

*AP = acid phosphate.

Medical Adrenalectomy

Various methods are available to block adrenal steroid synthesis chemically. If the exclusion of adrenal androgens is desired, these techniques offer an effective alternative to adrenalectomy as a means of further reducing circulating androgen levels after orchiectomy or estrogen treatment. Glucocorticoids, aminoglutethimide, and spironolactone have been used to counteract the production of adrenal androgens.

Glucocorticoids.—Glucocorticoids decrease adrenal androgen production indirectly by suppressing ACTH release. In a study by Miller and Hinman,[51] 8 of 10 patients who had relapsed after orchiectomy and received 50 mg of cortisone daily had subjective improvement with a mean duration of almost 3 months. In other studies,[50, 52] pain relief was reported in 14 of 16 (88%) treated patients. Tannock et al.[52] gave 10 mg of prednisone per day to 37 patients with refractory prostate cancer in a prospective fashion and monitored the subjective response carefully, including the use of several self-assessment scales. They found that 38% of the patients had an initial positive response, and that 19% of them maintained it for 3 to 30 months. This relief of pain was associated with a decrease in the level of adrenal androgens as well. It seems very possible that the majority of favorable subjective results with such therapy can be attributed to steroid-related euphoria, the anti-inflammatory activity of steroids, or other non-specific mechanisms of action, rather than to the decrease in adrenal androgen production. However, since the dose given by Tannock is below the Cushing threshold dose, the incidence of side effects is much lower and this treatment regimen may have a place in palliation.

Aminoglutethimide.—Aminoglutethimide blocks several cytochrome P-450–mediated hydroxylation reactions, including the conversion of cholesterol to pregnenolone and the hydroxylation of C-21, C-11, and C-18 steroids. The drug was introduced in 1960 as an anticonvulsant, but was removed from the market because of the development of adrenal insufficiency in some patients. It is given orally in a dose of 250 mg four times a day together with hydrocortisone to prevent adrenal insufficiency. Santen et al.[53] reviewed the reports available in the literature and found an overall response rate of 37.4% in 231 evaluable patients. Only 1% had a complete response, 13% had a partial response, and 4% had stabilization of their disease. In the only study that had used bidimensionally measurable lesions as an inclusion criterion,[54] no objective response was noted in 20 patients. Aminoglutethimide is also a powerful blocking agent of aromatase, the enzyme that is responsible for the synthesis of estradiol and estrone from testosterone and androstenedione. Considering the mechanisms of action of aminoglutethimide and hydrocortisone and the similarity of responses obtained with both agents, it is doubtful whether aminoglutithimide has any advantage over hydrocortisone alone.

Recently, Labrie et al.[55] reported on the use of aminoglutethimide plus low-dose glucocorticoids as third-line treatment in 119 patients who had failed castration and flutamide treatment. They found a significant difference in survival for 2 patients with a partial response and 15 patients with stable disease. This phase II study, however, is not suitable for comparing the differences in effectiveness, because the variability in survival between responders and nonresponders reflects the natural history of the disease rather than the effects of treatment.

Spironolactone.—Spironolactone inhibits adrenal and testicular cytochrome P-450 activity with resultant blockage of 17α-hydroxylase and 17,20-desmolase. It has been utilized as a means of medical adrenalectomy in only a few cases. Walsh and Siiteri[56] treated seven castrated men with metastatic and unresponsive prostate cancer with 100 and 400 mg of spironolactone per day and found a significant decline in testosterone, androstenedione, and dihydroepiandrosterone plasma levels. The major side effects of this treatment are hypercalcemia and gynecomastia.

Hypophysectomy and Pituitary Suppression

Hypophysectomy obviously will lead to the suppression of adrenal and testicular androgen production. Interference with testicular and adrenal pituitary feedback mechanisms, however, offers a more elegant mechanism with which to counteract androgen production selectively in these organs. Like adrenalectomy, early in the history of endocrine management of prostate cancer, hypophysectomy has been used as a means of second-line endocrine treatment in patients with progression after orchiectomy or testicular suppression. Estrogens commonly have been used to counteract luteinizing hormone and associated testosterone production. More elegantly, the recent advent of luteinizing hormone releasing hormone agonists and antagonists allows the selective suppression of luteinizing hormone production with virtually no estrogenic side effects. Some evidence exists[57] of a synergism between testosterone and prolactin in the hypophysectomized, castrated rat. This mechanism can be exploited for the treatment of prostate cancer by the use of prolactin inhibitors.

The first hypophysectomy for metastatic prostatic cancer was done in 1948 at the Johns Hopkins Hospital. The patient survived only 11 days. In 1962, Scott and Schirmer[58] reported a series of 60 patients who underwent open surgical hypophysectomy through a frontal craniotomy, resulting in subjective and objective remission in 7 of 10 evaluable patients. The results of hypophysectomy were reviewed by Brendler.[59] The theoretical advantage of hypophysectomy in the treatment of prostatic carcinoma is the elimination of the trophic stimuli caused by growth hormone, prolactin, ACTH, and luteinizing hormone. Several technical modalities for surgical removal of the pituitary gland are available. Despite some effectiveness as a second-line treatment, hypophysectomy does not play any role in the treatment of prostatic carcinoma at the present time.

Medical Control of Pituitary Hormone Production

Estrogens.—The first successful use of exogenous estrogens to treat prostate cancer was reported in 1942 by Herbst.[60] Since then, estrogens have been the most widely employed mode of hormonal therapy. They exert a variety of effects, the most important being the suppression of luteinizing hormone release from the pituitary by negative feedback. They also increase the production of sex-hormone−binding globulin, thereby decreasing the amount of available testosterone. Furthermore, estrogens interfere with the pituitary factor regulating prolactin production and lead to gynecomastia in men. Finally, estrogens inhibit 5α-reductase, interfere with the receptor binding of DHT and testosterone, inhibit DNA polymerase in the nucleus, and may have a direct toxic effect on the cancer cell. Specific evidence for the latter mechanism is scarce, but has been reviewed recently by van Steenbrugge.[61]

The most commonly used estrogens are synthetic preparations that are effective if taken orally. These include stilbene derivatives (diethylstilbestrol), estradiol esters (ethinyl estradiol, polyestradiol phosphate), and conjugated estrogens (Premarin). Diethylstilbestrol is the most widely used orally active estrogen preparation. It reliably reduces serum testosterone levels to castrate ranges at a dose of 3 mg daily, but may have an incomplete effect at 1 mg daily.[62−64] The use of 1 mg of diethylstilbestrol per day is associated with significantly fewer cardiovascular side effects. Despite the fact that it may not lower plasma testosterone to castration levels, it has been shown to be as effective as castration in protocol 30805 of the EORTC genitourinary group, which is a prospective randomized trial.[65]

A systemic attempt to study the effect of estrogens has been made by the Veterans Administration Cooperative Urological Research Group (VACURG). The first study of this group included patients with previously untreated stage C or D disease who were randomly assigned to receive either placebo, 5 mg of diethylstilbesterol daily, orchiectomy plus 5 mg of diethylstilbestrol, or orchiectomy plus placebo. Unfortunately, the trial methodology was suboptimal. Upon progression, patients in the placebo arm were moved to endocrine treatment and were still maintained in the original randomization scheme for evaluation. Therefore, the study in fact compares early vs. delayed endocrine management. Two findings are prominent: patients on placebo alone had a survival rate similar to the other groups, and patients on 5 mg of diethylstilbestrol had a higher mortality rate due to cardiovascular disease than did the other groups. Correct interpretation of the VACURG study allows the conclusion that early endocrine intervention did not increase survival when compared to delayed endocrine treatment in the placebo arm. Furthermore, 5 mg of diethylstilbestrol led to an increase in mortality and morbidity from cardiovascular complications.[66] Consequently, in the VACURG II study, patients were assigned to 5 mg of diethylstilbestrol vs. 1 mg vs. 0.2 mg daily. Both 5 mg and 1 mg daily were equally effective and superior to 0.2 mg daily with respect to survival.[67]

Chlorotrianisene (TACE) is also a stilbene derivative and has been used to treat metastatic prostate cancer. However, with the recommended dose of 12 mg daily, it produces only a 40% to 60% suppression of serum testosterone.[68] Another modality that can be used is diethylstilbestrol diphosphate (Stilphostrol) given as an intravenous high-dose infusion rescue therapy in refractory prostate cancer. Subjective (22%) and objective (70%) responses have been reported[69, 70] in patients with resistance to other forms of estrogen therapy. It is presumed that high doses of estrogens do have a direct cytotoxic effect on the prostate tumor cell. However, this has never been proven conclusively.

A compound that generated considerable interest, in particular in Europe, is estramustine phosphate (Emcyt), a combination of estrogen with nitrogen mustard connected in the form of a carbamate in the 3-position as a cytostatic agent. The original idea was to use the estrogen as a carrier to achieve high levels of cytotoxic drugs in the tumor itself and to prevent systemic toxicity. Despite considerable effort, it is not entirely clear whether the estrogen moiety alone, the nitrogen mustard moiety, or both together exert an antitumor effect. While estrogenic effects clearly do occur, it is also postulated that at the same time the drug has a cytostatic action. In a recent review of the literature by Anderson,[71] no differences in survival rates were reported with the use of estramustine phosphate in five prospective randomized trials in patients with previously untreated disease. In hormone-refractory patients, an average rate of response to therapy of 35% with a range of 0% to 74% is reported. Again, these data are based on a variety of patient selection and response criteria and do not establish the effectiveness of this drug beyond that of traditional estrogen treatment alone.

The NPCP as well as the EORTC genitourinary group have studied estrogen treatment in a prospective, randomized fashion. A recent review of the NPCP protocols is available by Elder and Gibbons.[72] A recent review of the EORTC genitourinary group studies has been done by Schröder.[73] This group compared 3 mg of diethylstilbestrol to estramustine phosphate, cyproterone acetate, and medroxyprogesterone acetate (EORTC protocols 30761 and 30762). One milligram of diethylstilbestrol was compared to orchiectomy and to orchiectomy plus cyproterone acetate 150 mg per day, a regimen that may be considered as total androgen suppression. No significant differences in progression-free and overall survival rates were seen, except for a worse outcome with medroxyprogesterone acetate, which was given at a relatively low dose. These studies were well conducted, analyzed prognostic factors, applied corrections accordingly, and reported side effects. They conclude that orchiectomy, orchiectomy plus cyproterone acetate, 3 mg of diethylstilbestrol, cyproterone acetate 250 mg per day, and 1 mg of diethylstilbestrol per day are equivalent treatments and differ only in side effects and complications.

Gestagens.—Megestrol acetate (Megace) and medroxyprogesterone acetate have been used in the management of patients with prostate cancer. These gestagens combine the features of estrogens in inhibiting pituitary luteinizing hormone release with the properties of classical antiandrogens, such as competitive binding to the androgen receptor with blockage of the 5α-reductase enzyme. Geller et al.[74] when treating 20 patients with 160 mg of megestrol acetate daily, noted that after an initial period of serum testosterone suppression, an escape phenomenon occurred and serum luteinizing hormone and testosterone levels started to rise again despite continued treatment. A possible explanation for this could be the direct antiandrogenic effect at the diencephalic target cells combined with an insufficient antigonadotropic effectiveness. Based on the late rise in serum testosterone, the authors recommended a trial combining megestrol acetate with low-dose diethylstilbestrol to prevent this undesirable effect. In EORTC protocol 30761, 200 mg of medroxyprogesterone acetate was inferior to diethylstilbestrol and cyproterone acetate as reported by Pavone-Macaluso et al.[16] Johnson[75] gave 160 mg of megestrol acetate in combination with 1 mg of diethylstilbestrol and found response rates similar to those obtained with 3 mg of diethylstilbestrol alone. An unexpectedly high incidence of side effects consisting of impotence, gynecomastia, lethargy, edema, and nausea was encountered.

Luteinizing Hormone Releasing Hormone Analogs.—In 1971, Schally et al.[76] discovered the decapeptide structure of the naturally occurring luteinizing hormone releasing hormone. Since then, over 2,000 of these analogs, agonists, and antagonists have been synthesized. Synthetic luteinizing hormone releasing hormone agonists with a substitution of D-leucine for glycine in position 6 are many times more powerful than the natural compound. By way of depletion of luteinizing hormone at the pituitary and down-regulation of luteinizing hormone releasing hormone receptors, after an initial rise, they lead to luteinizing hormone and testosterone suppression. Luteinizing hormone releasing hormone antagonists also have been synthesized, but despite the theoretical advantage of avoiding the initial rise in plasma testosterone levels, they have not been employed successfully in the management of human cancer.

The aforementioned properties make luteinizing hormone releasing hormone analogs suitable for monotherapy of hormone-responsive prostate cancer, especially if applied in depot preparations that lead to plasma testosterone suppression over 1 or several months. The initial rise in plasma testosterone can lead to an exacerbation of symptoms and maybe even early death.[77] This syndrome has been called the "flare phenomenon." The literature on flare has been reviewed recently by Boccon-Gibod.[78] The same author has described extensively the use of antiandrogens during the initial treatment period in prevention of the flare phenomenon. While the main mode of action of luteinizing hormone releasing hormone analogs is luteinizing hormone and plasma testosterone suppression, direct inhibition of tumor growth has been reported also.[79]

Several randomized prospective studies compared luteinizing hormone releasing hormone analogs in various regimens to standard treatment. The leuprolide study group[80] compared 3 mg of diethylstilbestrol to 1 mg of leuprolide daily. Parmar et al.[81] randomized long-acting D-tryptophan (Trp)-6-luteinizing hormone releasing hormone (LHRH)-microcapsules to orchiectomy in the second arm of a study conducted in previously untreated metastatic patients. No significant differences in progression and survival rates were encountered. In Parmar's study, three patients were reported to have significant flare. In the leuprolide study group, ten patients receiving leuprolide as compared to two receiving diethylstilbestrol had to be considered treatment failures because of progression prior to 3 months of therapy. Significant differences in response, progression, and survival rates were not reported. It can be expected that flare will severely affect only those patients with very advanced disease in critical locations (e.g., the spine or bones). In this respect, patient selection may be of crucial importance in applying luteinizing hormone releasing hormone analogs as monotherapy. The findings of these two studies were confirmed by Peeling et al.,[82] who compared a depot luteinizing hormone releasing hormone preparation (Zoladex) to 3 mg of diethylstilbestrol in 124 vs. 126 patients and, in a separate trial, to orchiectomy in 148 vs. 144 patients.

Luteinizing hormone releasing hormone analogs can be considered standard treatment provided flare is excluded by combining them with an antiandrogen during the first month of treatment. Side effects are limited to those of castration (hot flushes and gynecomastia). The question remains whether individuals and society are ready to pay for the much higher cost of this treatment in comparison to orchiectomy.

Prolactin Inhibition.—Experimental findings suggest that prolactin amplifies the effect of testosterone in the human prostate in some way[83] and thereby controls the growth of the organ to some degree. Jacobi[84] has found that not only serum prolactin levels but also serum testosterone levels fell after the administration of 15 mg of bromocriptine daily to 15 men with newly diagnosed prostate cancer, while luteinizing hormone and follicle-stimulating hormone levels remained unchanged. This was explained by a direct effect of bromocriptine on testicular testosterone secretion and a decrease in prolactin influencing the pituitary testicular axis. Furthermore, it was noted that the uptake of [^{3}H]-label by carcinoma tissue after the injection of 200 mCi of [^{3}H]-testosterone was decreased markedly after bromocriptine treatment. For unknown reasons, this effect was more pronounced in well-differentiated than in poorly differentiated tumor tissue. Jacobi[85] claims subjective and objective improvement using a low-dose estrogen treatment combined with bromocriptine in more than 50% of patients. This treatment has not been studied in a prospective randomized trial of sufficient size, and the treatment presently has no role as lone therapy of prostate cancer patients.

Antiandrogens

Antihormones are substances that counteract hormones at the target cell level rather than interfere with related feedback mechanisms. Antiandrogens probably exert their action by interfering with androgen binding to the androgen receptor. Because antiandrogens will affect all androgen-responsive and androgen-dependent target cells, they also will interfere with the androgen-regulated luteinizing hormone release in the pituitary. This is probably achieved by blocking androgen binding to receptor molecules in diencephalic luteinizing hormone releasing hormone—producing target cells. Since this is a negative feedback mechanism, the consequence is a rise in luteinizing hormone production and plasma testosterone.

A number of different antiandrogens are available. Figure 2 depicts the structural formulas of the most commonly used antiandrogens. Cyproterone acetate, because of its basic steroid hormone configuration and gesta-

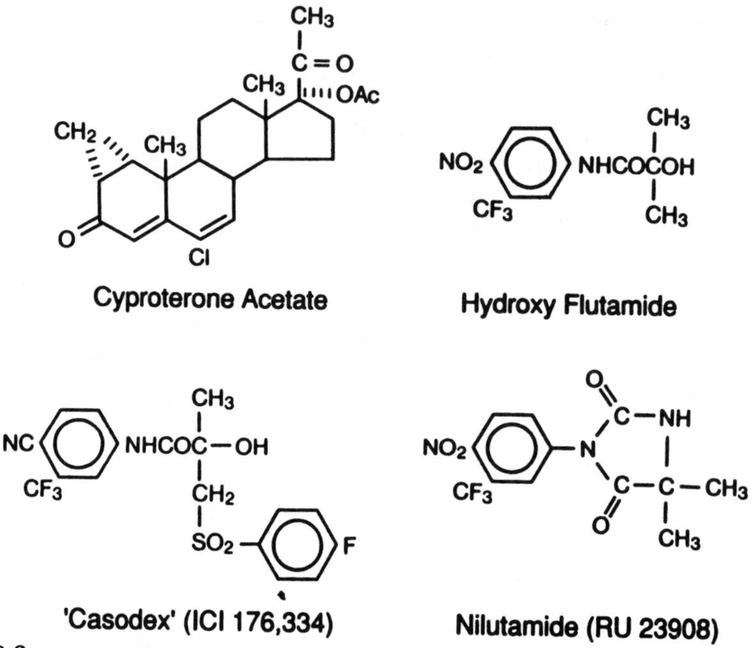

FIG 2.
Structural formulas of steroidal and nonsteroidal antiandrogens.

genic and antigonadotropic effects, is called a steroidal antiandrogen. Antiandrogens of the flutamide type are nonsteroidal or pure antiandrogens. The difference in endocrine effectiveness has been the subject of many comparative studies. Knuth and Nieschlag[86] studied young male volunteers over a period of 2 weeks. Their findings were similar to those of Neri, who compared cyproterone acetate and flutamide in the rat,[87] i.e., that cyproterone acetate reduces plasma testosterone and luteinizing hormone, but not to castration levels, while flutamide causes a rise in these levels. It is unknown whether this increase could lead to the stimulation of prostate cancer cell growth if pure antiandrogens are used as monotherapy for this disease. In a clinical study of 1 year's duration, Lund and Rasmussen[88] examined plasma testosterone values under flutamide monotherapy in comparison to diethylstilbestrol and found that after an initial rise lasting up to 6 months, plasma testosterone values decreased to about normal levels. Standard deviations, however, are very large in this limited experience with 20 patients. The pure antiandrogen casodex (ICI 167, 334) is more powerful than flutamide and has a longer half-life that allows oral administration once a day. The substance was claimed to be peripherally selective in the sense that it would not lead to a significant rise in plasma testosterone.[89] This assumption was based on experiments in animals that have not been reproduced in humans. In previously potent patients treated with pure antiandrogens, potency is usually preserved. This finding indicates a clinically relevant advantage if pure antiandrogen monotherapy could be shown to be as effective as standard forms of treatment. Some of the obvious endocrine effects of steroidal and nonsteroidal antiandrogens of the cyproterone acetate and flutamide type are shown in Table 4. Recent reviews of the most frequently used drugs and their basic properties are available in the literature.[89–92]

Cyproterone Acetate

As a steroidal antiandrogen, this compound is not only a competitive inhibitor of androgen binding to the receptor, but it also manifests progestational and antigonadotropic properties. It acts as a pituitary inhibitor and decreases luteinizing hormone and plasma testosterone, but not to castration levels. The drug has been used in monotherapy in several prospective randomized trials. Jacobi et al.[93] compared 300 mg of cyproterone acetate depot intramuscularly per week with 100 mg of estradiol undecylate depot intramuscularly per month in 203 patients. Short- and long-term results in both groups were very similar; no differences in response, progression, or survival were encountered. While gynecomastia, breast tenderness, and leg edema occurred in 77.1%, 78.5%, and 17.7%, respectively, of the estrogen treatment group, these side effects appeared in only 12.6%, 6.3%, and 4.2%, respectively, of the cyproterone acetate treatment group.

The EORTC compared 250 mg of cyproterone acetate per day in M0 and M1 patients in a prospective randomized study with 3 mg of diethylstilbestrol per day and 500 mg of intramuscular medroxyprogesterone acetate per day for 8 weeks followed by 200 mg orally per day as maintenance therapy.[16] A total of 210 eligible patients were entered between 1977 and 1981 and then followed until 1984 or death. A careful analysis

---

TABLE 4.
Effects of Steroidal and Nonsteroidal Antiandrogens on Endocrine Parameters

Endocrine Parameter	Nonsteroidal Antiandrogen (flutamide)	Steroidal Antiandrogen (cyproterone acetate)
Luteinizing hormone (plasma)	Increased	Decreased
Testosterone (plasma)	Increased	Decreased
Prostatic volume (rat and human)	Decreased*	Decreased
Seminal vesicle volume (rat)	Decreased*	Decreased
Libido	Unchanged	Decreased
Potency	Unchanged	Decreased

*Long-term effects not known in humans.

of prognostic factors was carried out. The results subsequently were used in the analysis of survival and progression data. This study established that cyproterone acetate is equivalent to standard treatment with diethylstilbestrol 3 mg per day. Furthermore, the study showed that these two regimens were superior to medroxyprogesterone acetate in the chosen dosage.

Flutamide

Flutamide is a nonsteroidal antiandrogen that probably acts by inhibiting the binding of testosterone and DHT to the androgen receptor in target tissues. Flutamide is also called a pure antiandrogen because, in contrast to cyproterone acetate, it does not possess any other endocrine activity. It has been found to be two times as potent as cyproterone acetate as an antiandrogen if used in castrate rats substituted with exogenous testosterone.[86] Considering its mechanism of action, it is obvious that flutamide does not suppress plasma testosterone levels; rather, these levels increase during treatment as a result of the lack of suppression of luteinizing hormone releasing hormone production at the level of the diencephalon and subsequently rising luteinizing hormone levels. Flutamide has no influence on adrenal androgen production.[94]

Flutamide has been studied as monotherapy in several phase II studies. Unfortunately, no sufficiently large phase III comparison to standard treatment has been carried out. The only comparative study (by Neri and Kassem[95]), which compared two different dosages of flutamide to diethylstilbestrol, has insufficient statistical power and follow-up to answer this question. Sogani[96] reported on 72 previously untreated stage D prostate cancer patients managed with 750 mg of flutamide, showing an overall 87.5% response. Unfortunately, follow-up is limited and progression and death rates are not known. Side effects of flutamide are gynecomastia and diarrhea. Potency is preserved in most previously potent patients. The effectiveness of flutamide as monotherapy in the management of prostate cancer patients has not been established in comparison to standard treatment.

The antiandrogen nilutamide is not recommended by the manufacturer for use in monotherapy. Casodex presently is being studied in phase II and III situations. Summaries of recent clinical findings are available in the literature.[97, 98]

Total Androgen Blockade

The concept of total androgen blockade has been applied in the past as a second-line endocrine treatment by eliminating adrenal androgens and/or pituitary stimulation. Labrie and his coworkers[99] advocated the principle of simultaneous exclusion of testicular and adrenal androgens as a primary form of management of patients with metastatic prostate cancer in 1983. They reported on 30 cases with an elevated acid phosphatase, of whom 29 reacted with a significant decrease of plasma enzyme levels. They concluded from their data that total androgen blockade as primary endocrine treatment was associated with a 97% response rate and that this management was superior to standard forms of treatment. The principle of total androgen blockade, however, had been applied previously in a phase III randomized study of metastatic, previously untreated prostate cancer patients by the EORTC genitourinary group in 1980.[65]

Theoretical Considerations

Clearly, the advantage of a potentially better and more effective form of treatment has to be established in clinical studies. Such studies are available now and will be referred to in the next section. This review shows that the data available at this moment are not entirely conclusive. However, sufficient information will be coming up shortly to answer directly the question whether total androgen blockade is superior to standard treatments such as orchiectomy.

During the phase of uncertainty about a possible superiority of total androgen blockade, a great wealth of experimental and preliminary clinical information has been produced. These arguments for and against total androgen blockade have been summarized recently by Labrie et al.[100] and Schröder and van Steenbrugge.[101] According to these publications, the theoretical advantage of total androgen blockade may be the further lowering of tissue androgen concentrations, which is indirect proof that adrenal androgens are metabolized to DHT. The demonstration of stimulation of growth by low androgen concentrations in some experimental systems, the variable sensitivity of clones of the Shionogi mammary tumor system to androgens, and the induction of heterogeneity of androgen responsiveness by low androgen levels have supplied additional arguments in favor of total androgen ablation. Arguments against any beneficial effect of eliminating adrenal androgens on prostate cancer are the lack of proliferative and functional response of human reproductive organs to adrenal androgens, the lack of stimulation of low androgen levels of the PC-82 human prostatic cancer line in nude mice, and the lack of stimulation of the well-established rat prostate cancer tumor line R-3327-H (Dunning tumor) by low concentrations of androgens. Labrie also maintains that the adrenal androgens dihydroepiandrosterone and androstenedione are converted in the prostate cell to testosterone and DHT, with the enzyme 17β-hydroxysteroid-dehydroxygenase playing a key role. This enzyme and its messenger RNA have been shown to be present in high concentrations in prostatic tissues.[55] Labrie presents evidence that after castration the DHT level in prostatic cancer tissue is about 40% of that in normal men. Only after combination therapy is no DHT detectable. Labrie does not offer an explanation as to why the addition of flutamide or luteinizing hormone releasing hormone agonist after castration reduces prostatic DHT to undetectable levels. This seems puzzling, since flutamide is supposed to inhibit the binding of DHT to the androgen receptor, but *not* the conversion of testosterone to DHT.

Total androgen blockade or suppression can be achieved in many different ways by combining treatment principles that achieve castration levels of plasma testosterone with an antiandrogen or by blocking steroidal genesis altogether. This can be achieved by primary hypophysectomy or by interfering with the cytochrome P-450 system of the C-17-20 liase responsible for the conversion of pregnenolone to 17-OH-progesterone (ketoconazole).

Clinical Application of Total Androgen Blockade

After a long and often heated debate about the possible theoretical advantages of total androgen suppression over standard endocrine treatment for metastatic prostate cancer, information is now becoming available from phase III studies that likely will give a definitive answer to this question within a year or two. No effort will be made in this context to review phase II studies and phase III studies that have insufficient statistical power to produce truly significant differences. Many of these studies, however, have one feature in common, a higher initial response rate with combination treatment. This probably was shown for the first time with solid data by Brisset and coworkers.[102]

The large phase III studies that are likely to give a definitive answer to the question regarding the superiority of total androgen suppression are summarized in Table 5. It is evident from this table that the results of very large, properly conducted studies at this moment are contradictory. While the National Cancer Institute study 0036, reported by Crawford et al.,[104] shows a significant difference in progression and survival rates in favor of the combination treatment in comparison to leuprolide alone, this difference is not reproduced by EORTC protocol 30843 comparing castration to busereline alone and busereline plus cyproterone acetate, or in the large international study comparing zoladex to zoladex plus flutamide in 568 patients. Despite the fact that a number of prospective randomized studies seem to indicate that luteinizing hormone releasing hormone monotherapy is equivalent to standard treatment, doubt has been expressed about the possibility that the flare phenomenon occurring with this therapy may have an impact on progression and survival.[78]

It is remarkable that none of the three large studies using castration as the control arm have shown an advantage in survival. In the Canadian study,[108] such an advantage was present previously, whereas progression rates were identical. The advantage in survival has disappeared prior to the latest report given at the annual meeting of the American Urological Association in 1990. EORTC protocol 30853 and the Danish Prostate Cancer Group (DAPROCA) study are virtually identical in patient selection and treatment schemes. A careful comparison of the distribution of prognostic factors has shown that a meta-analysis is feasible, and this has been carried out. It shows that the difference in progression rates in favor of the combination treatment persists, and that a difference in survival is not seen. However, it must be stated that in some of the studies cited,[103, 105, 106, 108] median time to progression and median survival have not yet been reached. These data need to mature further to allow definitive conclusions.

From the available evidence, it can be concluded that daily injections of 1 mg of leuprolide in combination with 750 mg of flutamide as compared

TABLE 5.
Summary of Results of Phase III Studies Employing Total Androgen Blockade (M0-1 Patients, Previously Untreated)*

Author	Design	Number of Patients	Preliminary Outcome
Haldaway et al.[103]	Zoladex vs. zoladex and flutamide	568	Not significant (survival, progression)
Crawford et al.[104] (NCI 0036)	Leuprolide vs. leuprolide and flutamide	603	Survival and progression better (P < .05) for combination arm
de Voogt et al.[105] (EORTC 30843)	Castration vs. busereline vs. busereline and cyproterone acetate	367	Not significant, survival and progression (preliminary data)
Keuppens et al.[106] (EORTC 30853)	Zoladex vs. castration and flutamide	327	Progression better for combination, survival not significant
Iversen et al.[107] (DAPROCA)	Zoladex vs. castration and flutamide	264	Progression and survival not significant
Trachtenberg et al.[108] (Canadian study)	Castration vs. castration and anandron	203	Progression and survival not significant

*NCI = National Cancer Institute; EORTC = European Organization for Research on Treatment of Cancer; DAPROCA = Danish Prostate Cancer Group.

to leuprolide alone are associated with a significant advantage in progression and survival rates. This advantage amounts to differences of 2.6 months in median time to progression and 7.3 months in median survival. These differences are not reproduced by the preliminary results of studies using castration as the standard treatment control arm. At this moment, therefore, there seems to be insufficient evidence to recommend total androgen blockade as standard treatment in all patients with metastatic prostate cancer. The size of the available studies does not allow a significant subgroup analysis to identify those patients that may benefit most from combination treatment, although evidence from the Leuprolide Study Group suggests that patients with good performance status benefit more from combination treatment.

Unresolved Issues in Endocrine Management of Prostate Cancer

Despite a very large volume of clinical studies, the question whether endocrine management prolongs the survival of patients with metastatic prostate cancer is still unresolved. The VACURG studies suggest that this may not be the case. However, considering the poor design of these studies, confirmation is necessary. Furthermore, it remains unresolved whether there is an advantage to early or delayed endocrine management. Again, the VACURG studies are the only ones addressing this problem. The results suggest that delay of treatment until symptoms of metastatic disease occur is not associated with a shorter life span. A recent study by Myers et al.[109] suggests that there may be a significant difference in favor of early endocrine treatment provided the patient's primary tumor is shown to be diploid. This holds true, however, only for patients with a limited volume of metastases (N1-2 disease). The EORTC genitourinary group presently is studying this problem (protocol 30846).

Since endocrine treatment is palliative at best, and since it is doubtful whether this management is associated with an advantage in survival, treatment modalities that are associated with the fewest side effects should have priority. In this respect, the maintenance of libido and potency is a relevant issue. It is necessary to study prospectively, in randomized studies, using standard treatment in the control arm, the long-term use of pure antiandrogens and perhaps also 5α-reductase inhibitors as monotherapy.

There are suggestions in studies by Myers[109] and others that there is a group of patients that does not benefit from endocrine treatment at all. If these patients could be identified at the time of diagnosis, they probably should not be treated by endocrine means. Finally, it should not be forgotten that nearly all patients with metastatic prostate cancer finally suffer progression to a hormone-independent tumor that eventually will lead to death, irrespective of endocrine treatment. Therefore, the highest priority in the management of prostate cancer is the search for effective treatment of hormone-unresponsive disease.

References

1. Coffey DS, Isaacs JT: Control of prostate growth. *Urology* 1981; 3:17–24.
2. Lipsett B: Interaction of drugs, hormones and nutrition in the causes of cancer. *Cancer* 1979; 43:1967–1981.
3. Yatani R, Chigusa I, Akazaki K, et al: Geographic pathology of latent prostatic carcinoma. *Int J Cancer* 1982; 29:611–616.
4. Akazaki K, Stemmerman GN: Comparative study of latent carcinoma of the prostate among Japanese in Japan and Hawaii. *J Natl Cancer Inst* 1973; 50:1137–1144.
5. Hänäläinen E, Aldercreutz H, Puska P, et al: Diet and serum sex hormones in healthy men. *J Steroid Biochem* 1984; 20:459–464.
6. de Jong FH, Oishi K, Hayes RB, et al: Peripheral hormone levels in controls and patients with prostatic cancer or benign prostatic hyperplasia: Results from the Dutch-Japanese case-control study. Submitted for publication.
7. Coffey DS, Pietna KJ: New concepts in studying the control of normal and cancer growth of the prostate. *Prog Clin Biol Res* 1987; 239:1–73.
8. Tilley WD, Marcelli M, Wilson JD, et al: Characterization and expression of a cDNA encoding the human androgen receptor. *Proc Natl Acad Sci USA* 1989; 86:327–331.
9. Huggins C, Stevens RE, Hodges CV: Studies in prostatic cancer II. The effects of castration on advanced carcinoma of the prostate gland. *Arch Surg* 1941; 43:209.
10. Isaacs JT, Wake N, Coffey DS, et al: Genetic instability coupled to clonal selection as a mechanism for tumor progression in the Dunning R-3327 rat prostatic adenocarcinoma system. *Cancer Res* 1982; 42:2353–2361.
11. Oesterling JE, Epstein JI, Walsh PC: The viability of adrenal androgens to stimulate the adult human prostate: An autopsy, evaluation of men with hypogonadotropic hypogonadism and panhypopituitarism. *J Urol* 1986; 136:1030–1034.
12. Isaacs JT, Kyprianou N: Development of androgen independent tumor cells and their implication for the treatment of prostatic cancer. *Urol Res* 1987; 15:133–138.
13. Murphy GP, Slack NH: Response criteria to the prostate of the USA National Prostatic Cancer Project. *Prostate* 1980; 1:375–382.
14. Schröder FH, European Organization for Research on Treatment of Cancer, Urological Group: Treatment response criteria for prostatic cancer. *Prostate* 1984; 5:181–191.
15. Newling DWW: Criteria of response to treatment in advanced prostatic cancer. *Baillieres Clin Oncol* 1988; 2:505–519.
16. Pavone-Maculso M, de Voogt HJ, Viggiano G, et al: Comparison of diethylstilbestrol, cyproterone acetate, medroxyprogesterone acetate in the treatment of advanced prostatic cancer: Final analysis of a randomized phase II trial of the European Organization for Research on Treatment. *J Urol* 1986; 136:624–631.
17. Smith PH, Suciu S, Robinson MRG, et al: A comparison of the effect of diethylstilbestrol with low dose estramustine phosphate in the treatment of advanced prostatic cancer: Final analysis of a phase III trial of the European Organization for Research on Treatment of Cancer. *J Urol* 1986; 136:619–623.
18. Carpentier PJ, Schröder FH: Transrectal ultrasonography in the follow-up of

prostatic carcinoma patients: A new prognostic parameter? *J Urol* 1984; 131:903–905.

19. Carpentier PJ, Schröder FH, Schmitz PIM: Transrectal ultrasonometry of the prostate: The prognostic relevance of volume changes under endocrine management. *World J Urol* 1986; 44:159–162.

20. Sneller ZW, Carpentier PJ, Hop WC, et al: Prognostic value of prostatic volume reduction in the endocrine management of prostatic carcinoma (abstract). *J Urol* 1990; 143:308A.

21. Isaacs JT: Antagonistic effect of androgen on prostatic cell death. *Prostate* 1984; 5:545–557.

22. Montpetit ML, Lawless KR, Tenniswood M: Androgen-repressed message in the rat ventral prostate. *Prostate* 1986; 8:25–36.

23. Humphries JE, Isaacs JT: Unusual androgen sensitivity of the androgen independent Dunning R3327-G rat prostatic adenocarcinoma: Androgen effect on tumor cell loss. *Cancer Res* 1982; 42:3148–3156.

24. Habib FK, Lee IR, Stitch SR, et al: Androgen levels in the plasma and prostatic tissues of patients with benign hypertrophy and carcinoma of the prostate. *J Endocrinol* 1976; 7:99–107.

25. Ghanadian R, Puah CM: Relationship between oestradiol-17-beta, testosterone, dehydrotestosterone and 5-alpha-androstane-3-alpha, 17-beta-diol in human benign hypertrophy and carcinoma of the prostate. *J Endocrinol* 1981; 88:255–262.

26. Geller J, Albert JD, Loza D, et al: DHT concentrations in human prostate cancer tissue. *J Clin Endocrinol Metab* 1978; 46:440–444.

27. Krieg M, Bartsch W, Janssen W, et al: A comparative study of binding, metabolism and endogenous levels of androgens in normal, hyperplastic and carcinomatous human prostate, in Coffey DS, Isaacs JT, (eds): *Prostate Cancer*. Geneva, UICC Technical Report Series 48, 1979, pp 93–111.

28. Siiteri PK, Wilson JD: The formation and content of dehydrotestosterone in the hypertrophic prostate of man. *J Clin Invest* 1970; 49:1737–1745.

29. Walsh PC, Hutchins GM, Ewing LL: Tissue content of dehydrotestosterone in human prostatic hyperplasia is not supranormal. *J Clin Invest* 1983; 72:1772–1777.

30. Bolton NJ, Lukkarinen O, Vikho R: Concentrations of androgens in human benign prostatic hypertrophic tissues incubated for up to three days. *Prostate* 1986; 9:159–167.

31. Labrie F, Veilleux R, Fournier A: Low androgen levels induce the development of androgen-hypersensitive cell clones in Shionogi mouse mammary carcinoma cells in culture. *J Natl Cancer Inst* 1988; 80:1138–1147.

32. van Weerden WM, van Steenbrugge GJ, van Kreuningen A, et al: Assessment of the critical level of androgen for growth response of transplantable human prostatic carcinoma (PC-82) in nude mice. *J Urol* 1991; in press.

33. van Steenbrugge GJ: *Transplantable Human Prostate Cancer (PC-82) in Athymic Nude Mice: A Model for the Study of Androgen-Regulated Tumor Growth (thesis)*. Erasmus University, Rotterdam, 1988.

34. Labrie F, Belanger A, Veilleux R, et al: Rationale for maximal androgen withdrawal in the therapy of prostate cancer. *Baillieres Clin Oncol* 1988; 2:597–618.

35. Petrow V, Padilla GM, Mukherji S, et al: Endocrine dependence of prostatic cancer upon dihydrotestosterone and not upon testosterone. *J Pharm Pharmacol* 1984; 36:352–353.

36. Huggins C, Hodges CV: Studies on prostate cancer. I. The effect of castra-

tion, of estrogen and of androgen injection on serum phosphatases in metastatic carcinoma of the prostate. *Cancer Res* 1941; 1:293–297.
37. Robinson MRG, Thomas BS: Effect of hormonal therapy on plasma testosterone levels in prostatic carcinoma. *Br Med J [Clin Res]* 1971; 4:391–394.
38. Riba LW: Subcapsular castration for carcinoma of prostate. *J Urol* 1942; 48:384–387.
39. Clark P, Houghton L: Subcapsular orchiectomy for carcinoma of the prostate. *Br J Urol* 1977; 49:419–425.
40. Senge T, Hulshoff T, Tunn U, et al: Testosteron Konzentration in Serum nach subkapsulaerer Orchiektomie. *Urologe [A]* 1978; 17:382–384.
41. Huggins C, Wallace Scott W: Bilateral adrenalectomy in prostatic cancer. Clinical features and urinary excretion of 17-ketosteroids and estrogen. *Ann Surg* 1945; 122:1031–1041.
42. West CD, Hollander VP, Whitmore WF, et al: The effect of bilateral adrenalectomy upon neoplastic disease in man. *Cancer* 1952; 5:1009–1018.
43. Harrison JH, Thorn GW, Jenkins D: Total adrenalectomy for reactivated carcinoma of the prostate. *N Engl J Med* 1953; 248:86–91.
44. Baker WJ: Bilateral adrenalectomy for carcinoma of the prostate gland: Preliminary report. *J Urol* 1953; 70:275–281.
45. Scardino PL, Prince CL, McGoldrick ThA: Bilateral adrenalectomy for prostatic cancer. *J Urol* 1953; 70:100–109.
46. Taylor SG, Li MC, Eckles N, et al: Effect of surgical Addison's disease on advanced carcinoma of the breast and prostate. *Cancer* 1953; 6:997–1009.
47. Morales PA, Brendler H, Hotchkiss RS: The role of the adrenal cortex in prostatic cancer. *J Urol* 1955; 73:399–409.
48. MacFarlane DA, Thomas LP, Harrison JH: A survey of total adrenalectomy in cancer of the prostate. *Am J Surg* 1960; 99:562–572.
49. Schoonees R, Schalch DS, Reynoso G, et al: Bilateral adrenalectomy for advanced prostatic carcinoma. *J Urol* 1972; 108:123–125.
50. Mahony EM, Hartwell Harrison J: Bilateral adrenalectomy for palliative treatment of prostatic cancer. *J Urol* 1972; 108:936–938.
51. Miller GM, Hinman F: Cortisone treatment in advanced carcinoma of the prostate. *J Urol* 1954; 72:485–496.
52. Tannock I, Gospodarowic M, Meakin W, et al: Treatment of metastatic prostatic cancer with low-dose prednisone: Evaluation of pain and quality of life as pragmatic indices of response. *J Clin Oncol* 1989; 7:590–597.
53. Santen RJ, English H, Rohner T, et al: Androgen depletion/repletion in combination with chemotherapy: Strategy for secondary treatment of metastatic prostatic cancer, in Schröder FH, Richards B (eds): *EORTC GU Group Monograph 2, Part A: Therapeutic Principles in Metastatic Prostatic Cancer.* New York, Alan Liss Inc, pp 359–371.
54. Block M, Trump D, Rose DP, et al: Evaluation of aminogluthemide in stage D prostate cancer. *Cancer Treat Res* 1984; 68:719–722.
55. Labrie F, Dupont A, Belanger A, et al: Antihormone treatment for prostate cancer relapsing after treatment with flutamide and castration. *Br J Urol* 1989; 63:634–638.
56. Walsh PC, Siiteri PK: Suppression of plasma androgens by spironolactone in castrated men with carcinoma of the prostate. *J Urol* 1975; 114:254–256.
57. Grayhack JT, Bunce PL, Kearns JW, et al: Influence of the pituitary on prostatic response to androgen in the rat. *Bull Johns Hopkins Hosp* 1955; 96:154–163.

58. Scott WW, Schirmer HKA: Hypophysectomy for disseminated prostatic cancer, in Boyland E (ed): *On Cancer and Hormones: Essays in Experimental Biology*, Chicago, University of Chicago Press, 1966, p 175.
59. Brendler H: Adrenalectomy and hypophysectomy for prostatic cancer. *Urology* 1973; 2:99–102.
60. Herbst WP: Biochemical therapeusis in carcinoma of the prostate gland. *JAMA* 1942; 120:1116–1122.
61. van Steenbrugge GJ, Groen M, van Kreuningen A, et al: Transplantable human prostatic carcinoma (PC-82) in athymic nude mice. III. Effects of estrogens on the growth of the tumor tissue. *Prostate* 1988; 12:157–171.
62. Prout Jr GR, Kliman B, Daly JJ, et al: Endocrine changes after diethylstilbestrol therapy. Effects in prostatic neoplasm and pituitary gonadal axis. *Urology* 1976; 7:148–155.
63. Shearer RJ, Hendry WF, Sommerville IF, et al: Plasma testosterone an accurate monitor of hormone treatment in prostatic cancer. *Br J Urol* 1973; 45:668–677.
64. Beck PH, McAnich JW, Goebel JL, et al: Plasma testosterone in patients receiving DES. *Urology* 1978; 11:157–160.
65. Robinson MRG, Hetherington J: The EORTC studies: Is there an optimal endocrine management for MI prostatic cancer? *World J Urol* 1986; 4:1–5.
66. Blackard CE, Byar DP, Jordan WP: Orchiectomy for advanced prostatic carcinoma. *Urology* 1973; 1:553–560.
67. Bailar JC, Byar DP: Estrogen treatment for cancer of the prostate. Early results with three doses of DES and placebo. *Cancer* 1970; 26:257–261.
68. Baba S, Janetschek G, Pollow K, et al: The effect of chlorotrianise (TACE) on kinetics of 3H-testosterone in metabolism in patients with carcinoma of the prostate. *Br J Urol* 1982; 54:393–398.
69. Citrin DL, Kies MS, Wallemark CB, et al: A phase II study of high-dose estrogens (diethylstilbestrol diphosphate) in prostate cancer. *Cancer* 1985; 56:457–460.
70. Band PR, Banerjee TK, Patwardhan VC, et al: High-dose diethylstilbestrol diphosphate therapy of prostatic cancer after failure of standard doses of estrogens. *Can Med Assoc J* 1973; 109:697–699.
71. Andersson L: Estrogens and estramustine phosphate, in Denis L (ed): *The Medical Management of Prostate Cancer*. Heidelberg, Springer-Verlag, 1988, pp 37–42.
72. Elder JS, Gibbons RP: Results of trials of the USA National Prostatic Cancer Project, in Schroeder FH, Richards B (eds): *EORTC Genitourinary Group Monograph 2, Part A: Therapeutic Principles in Metastatic Prostatic Cancer*. New York, Alan Liss, 1985, pp 221–242.
73. Schröder FH: EORTC Genitourinary Group: Prostate cancer studies, in Schröder FH(ed): *EORTC Genitourinary Group Monograph: Treatment of Prostatic Cancer: Facts and Controversies*. New York, Alan Liss, 1990.
74. Geller J, Albert J, Yen SSC: Treatment of advanced cancer of prostate with megestrol acetate. *Urology* 1978; 12:537–541.
75. Johnson DE, Babaian RJ, Swanson DA, et al: Medical castration using megestrol acetate and minidose estrogen. *Urology* 1988; 31:371–374.
76. Schally AV, Arimura A, Baba Y, et al: Isolation and properties of the FSH and LH-releasing hormone. *Biochem Biophys Res Commun* 1971; 43:393–399.
77. Schroeder FH, Lock MTWT, Chadha DR, et al: Metastatic cancer of the

prostate managed with buserelin versus buserelin plus cyproterone acetate. *J Urol* 1987; 137:912–918.

78. Boccon-Gibod L: The prevention of LHRH induced disease flare in patients with metastatic carcinoma of the prostate, in Schroeder FH (ed): *EORTC Genitourinary Group Monograph: Treatment of Prostatic Cancer: Facts and Controversies.* New York, Alan Liss, 1990, pp 125–130.

79. Ostensen R: Direct effects of the LHRH agonist D-Leu-6-LHRH on human prostate carcinoma cell lines: Presence of a specific binding protein in vitro inhibition (abstract). *Am Fed Clin Res* 1986.

80. Leuprolide Study Group: Leuprolide versus diethylstilbestrol for metastatic prostate cancer. *N Engl J Med* 1984; 311:1281–1286.

81. Parmar H, Lightman SL, Allen L, et al: Randomised controlled study of orchidectomy versus long-acting D-TRP-6-LHRH microcapsules in advanced prostatic carcinoma. *Lancet* 1985; 8466:1201–1205.

82. Peeling WB: Phase III studies to compare goserelin (Zoladex) with orchiectomy and DES in treatment of prostatic carcinoma. *Urology* 1989; 33:45–51.

83. Farnsworth WE, Slaunwhite WR, Sharma M, et al: Interaction of prolactin and testosterone in the human prostate. *Urol Res* 1981; 9:79–88.

84. Jacobi GH, Sinterhauf K, Kurth KH, et al: Bromocriptine and prostatic carcinoma: Plasma kinetics, production and tissue uptake of 3H-testosterone in vivo. *J Urol* 1978; 119:240–243.

85. Jacobi GH: *Palliativtherapie des Prostatakarzinomas. Endokrinologische Grundlagen, klinische Situation, Prolaktin—ein neues Prinzip.* Muenchen, Zuckschwerdt, 1980.

86. Knuth UA, Hano R, Nieschlag E: Effect of flutamide or cyproterone acetate on pituitary and testicular hormones in normal men. *J Clin Endocrinol Metab* 1984; 59:963–969.

87. Neri RO, Florance K, Koziol P, et al: A biological profile of a nonsteroidal antiandrogen SCH-13521 (4'-nitro-3'-trifluoromethylisobutyranilide). *Endocrinology* 1972; 91:427–437.

88. Lund F, Rasmussen F: Flutamide versus stilbestrol in the management of advanced prostatic cancer. *Br J Urol* 1988; 61:140–142.

89. Furr BJA: The case for pure antiandrogens. *Baillieres Clin Oncol* 1988; 2:581–590.

90. Jacobi GH, Neumann F: The case for cyproterone acetate. *Baillieres Clin Oncol* 1988; 2:571–580.

91. Ojasoo T: Nilutamide. *Drugs of the Future* 1987; 12:763–770.

92. Neri RO: Studies on the biology and mechanism of action of nonsteroidal antiandrogens, in Martini L, Motta M (eds): *Androgens and Antiandrogens.* New York, Raven Press, 1977, pp 179–189.

93. Jacobi GH, Altwein JE, Kurth KH, et al: Treatment of advanced prostatic cancer with parenteral cyproterone acetate: A phase III randomised trial. *Br J Urol* 1980; 52:208–215.

94. Hellman L, Bradlow HL, Freed S, et al: The effect of flutamide on testosterone metabolism and the plasma levels of androgens and gonadotropins. *J Clin Endocrinol Metab* 1977; 45:1224–1229.

95. Neri RO, Kassem NY: Biological and clinical properties of antiandrogens. *Prog Cancer Res Ther* 1984; 31:507–518.

96. Sogani PC, Minoo R, Vagaiwala R, et al: Experience with flutamide in patients with advanced prostatic cancer without prior endocrine therapy. *Cancer* 1984; 54:744–750.

97. Schroeder FH: Pure antiandrogens as monotherapy in prospective studies of prostatic carcinoma, in Schroeder FH (ed): *EORTC Genitourinary Group Monograph: Treatment of Prostatic Cancer: Facts and Controversies.* New York, Alan Liss, 1990, pp 93–104.
98. Pavone-Macaluso M, Pavone M, Serretta V, et al: Antiandrogens alone or in combination for treatment of prostate cancer: The European experience. *Urology* 1989; 34(suppl 4):27–36.
99. Labrie F, Dupont A, Belanger A, et al: New approaches in the treatment of prostate cancer: Complete instead of partial withdrawal of androgens. *Prostate* 1983; 4:579–594.
100. Labrie F, Belanger A, Veilleux R, et al: Rationale for maximal androgen withdrawal in the therapy of prostate cancer. *Baillieres Clin Oncol* 1988; 2:597–619.
101. Schroeder FH, van Steenbrugge GJ: Rationale against total androgen withdrawal. *Baillieres Clin Oncol* 1988; 2:621–633.
102. Brisset JM, Boccon-Gibod L, Botto H, et al: Anandron (RU 23908) associated to surgical castration in previously untreated stage D prostate cancer: A multicenter comparative study of two doses of the drug and of a placebo, in Khoury S, Murphy GP (eds): *Prostate Cancer.* New York, Alan Liss, 1987, pp 411–422.
103. Haldaway I, Altwein JE, Klippel KF, et al: A multicenter randomised trial comparing the LHRH agonist Zoladex with Zoladex in combination with flutamide in the treatment of advanced prostate cancer (abstract). *J Urol* 1990; 143:220A.
104. Crawford ED, Eisenberger MA, McLeod DG, et al: A controlled trial of leuprolide with and without flutamide in prostatic carcinoma. *N Engl J Med* 1989; 321:419–424.
105. de Voogt HJ, Klijn JGM, Studer U, et al: Orchiectomy versus buserelin in combination with cyproterone acetate for 2 weeks or continuously in the treatment of metastatic prostatic cancer. Submitted for publication.
106. Keuppens F, Denis L, Smith PH, et al: Zoladex R and flutamide versus bilateral orchiectomy: A randomized phase III EORTC 30853 study. *Cancer,* 1990; 66:39–51.
107. Iversen P, Suciu S, Sylvester R, et al: Zoladex and flutamide versus orchiectomy in the treatment of advanced prostatic cancer. A combined analysis of two European studies—EORTC 30853 and DAPROCA 86. *Cancer* 1990; 66:52–66.
108. Trachtenberg J, personal communication, 1990.
109. Myers RP, Oesterling JE, Zincke H, et al: Critical association of DNA ploidy and prognosis of stage D1 prostate cancer patients treated with radical prostatectomy and early or delayed endocrine therapy (abstract). *J Urol* 1990; 143:712.

Cavitron Resection (Ultrasonic Aspiration) of the Prostate

Terrence R. Malloy, M.D.

Professor of Urology, University of Pennsylvania School of Medicine,
Philadelphia, Pennsylvania

Ultrasonic aspiration of the tissue was first made possible by the invention of the solid acoustic horn by Mason. This device converted electrical energy into mechanical motion at the tip of a hollow titanium cylinder that vibrated longitudinally along its axis at ultrahigh frequencies. von Ardeene and Grossman in 1960 first reported the removal of tissue with hollow ultrasonically vibrating needles.[1] In 1967, Banko and Kelman[2] developed phacoemulsifier for cataract extraction. Flamm and colleagues reported ultrasonic aspiration of neurogenic tumors in 1978.[3] Subsequently, Hodgson in 1979 reported on an ultrasonic scalpel for liver surgery.[4]

In urology, Addonizio and associates first described the ultrasonic aspira-

---

TABLE 1.
Technical Specifications

I. Functional components.
  A. Endoscopic sheath—26.5 F.
  B. Telescope—12-F, 90-degree field of view inclined at 45 degrees.
  C. Ultrasonic tip—12-F bore, titanium alloy metal.
  D. Irrigation—glycine.
  E. Aspiration—100 to 760 mm Hg inlet pressure.
  F. Cautery—ultrasonic tip connected to standard electrosurgical generator that may be applied independently or simultaneously with ultrasonic vibration.
II. Performance.
  A. Ultrasonic tip—0 to 700 μm vibration level at excursion rate of 39 kHz adjustable.
  B. Ultrasonic power—100-W maximum.
  C. Tissue dissection rate—1 to 3 g/min of prostatic adenoma.
  D. Irrigation—200 cc/min over telescopic lens gravity fed at 200 cm pressure.
  E. Aspiration—free fluid at 1 L/min at 300 mm Hg inlet pressure.

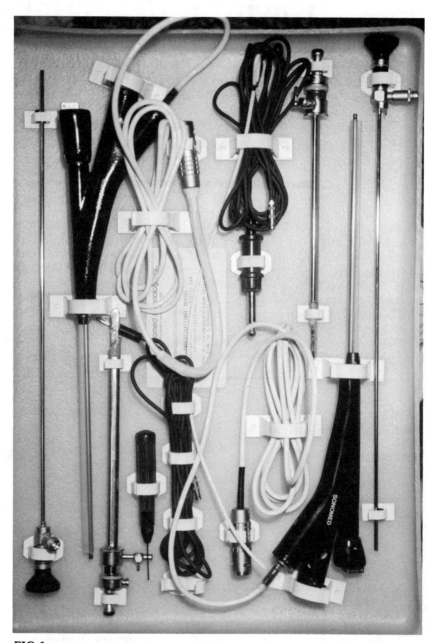

FIG 1.
The ultrasonic aspirator equipment consisting of the sheath, telescope, and titanium ultrasonic aspirator.

tor in renal surgery in 1983.[5-7] Essentially used for renal parenchymal surgery, the device had limited use except in partial nephrectomies. It was 1986 before Wuchinich devised an endoscopic ultrasonic aspirator that could be utilized transurethrally to remove prostatic adenoma. The device produced by Wuchinich (Fig 1) is unique in combining fragmentation, irrigation, and aspiration simultaneously. Tissue high in water content (prostate adenoma) is fragmented selectively while sparing collagen-laden tissue such as the prostatic capsule, bladder neck, and external sphincter. Initial reports by Malloy and associates in 1989 regarding the efficacy of this treatment were encouraging.[8] Technical specifications for the endoscopic ultrasonic aspirator are listed in Table 1.

Study Group

Commencing in June 1988, at the Pennsylvania Hospital of the University of Pennsylvania, a study to assess the feasibility of transurethral ultrasonic aspiration of the prostate was undertaken in males afflicted with bladder outlet obstruction, presumably due to benign prostatic hyperplasia. Patients were selected on the basis of symptoms and history.

Preoperative Evaluation

Preoperative evaluation included an intravenous pyelogram or ultrasound of the kidneys, complete urodynamics (CMG, flow, and urethral pressure profile), cystoscopy, laboratory evaluation (complete blood count, SMA-12, peroxidase-antiperoxidase test, and prostate-specific antigen test), and urinalysis with urine culture and sensitivity.

Patient Assessment

All patients to be considered for ultrasonic aspiration of the prostate were evaluated clinically to prove bladder outlet obstruction from an enlarged prostate. An intravenous pyelogram or ultrasound of the kidneys was used to assess upper tract competence and function. Complete urodynamics were performed to rule out irritative or dysfunctional voiding symptoms, neurogenic bladder, or atonic bladder. Patients to be considered for this surgery were required to have a maximum flow rate of less than 8 mL/sec and a mean flow of less than 5 mL/sec. Cystoscopy was performed to evaluate the size and nature of the obstruction from the prostatic adenoma. Stricture disease was ruled out also. In addition, prostatic-specific antigen and acid phosphatase were performed to rule out obvious carcinomas.

All patients signed an informed consent form since endoscopic ultrasonic aspiration of the prostate is not approved by the U.S. Food and Drug Administration at this time. The patients were assured that if problems arose during the procedure, the operation would be completed by a standard electrocautery transurethral resection of the prostate. The patients also were informed that at the termination of the endoscopic aspiration, transurethral resection biopsies of each lateral lobe would be performed to compare pathology between ultrasonically aspirated and electrocautery-resected tissue.

Surgical Technique

All patients had the usual preoperative surgical assessment with appropriate laboratory and blood studies performed. Anesthesia was administered by spinal or general means. Cystoscopy was performed to reassess the size and configuration of the prostatic adenoma. Urethral sounds were passed to 28 F to assure easy passage of the endoscopic ultrasonic sheath. The ultrasonic aspirator was introduced with a 12-French 12-degree telescope through a 26.5-F sheath. Glycine was utilized for irrigation. A cautery attachment was put in place at the base of the instrument (Fig 2).

The initial aspiration was commenced at the most distal portion of each lateral lobe. The principal difference in technique between ultrasonic aspiration and transurethral resection of the prostate is that the instrument is

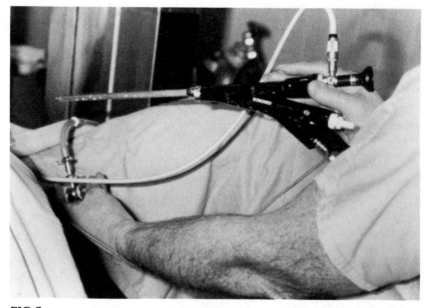

FIG 2.
The ultrasonic aspirator is introduced into the sheath, which is already inserted into the bladder. Electrocautery is attached to the base of the instrument as well as to the aspirating tube.

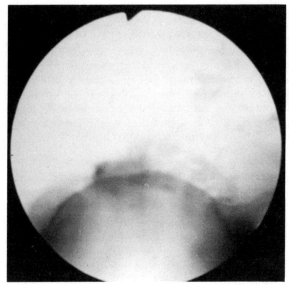

FIG 3.
Endoscopic view of the hollow core aspirator being introduced retrogradely into the prostatic adenoma.

moved into the tissue in a retrograde fashion with ultrasonic aspiration (Fig 3). The hollow core presses into the tissue, fragmenting and aspirating it simultaneously. When bleeding vessels were encountered, electrocautery was passed down the hollow core, which was laid against the vessels for coagulation. When both lateral lobes had been removed by aspiration, the middle and anterior lobes were treated simultaneously. Aspiration can proceed routinely at a rate of between 1 and 3 g/min. At the completion of the procedure, there was no need for removal of tissue, since it had been aspirated continually during the surgery. A resectoscope was introduced into the bladder and biopsies were taken of both lateral lobes for comparative pathology. When this ultrasonic aspiration technique is approved by the Food and Drug Administration, this will not be necessary any longer. A Foley catheter was left in place for 18 to 24 hours. The patients were discharged routinely from the hospital on the second or third postoperative day.

Results

Forty men have been followed for more than 18 months or longer after ultrasonic aspiration of the prostate. Blood loss has been minimal, with no transfusions required. There were no changes in postoperative electrolytes or renal function in any of the patients. All men voided satisfactorily when the catheters were removed and none experienced secondary bleeding in the immediate postoperative period. Thirty-seven men had benign prostatic hyperplasia on both aspirated and transurethral resection specimens, while 3 had adenocarcinoma on both tissue samples.

In 28 of 40 males active sexually after ultrasonic aspiration, 23 (82%) had antegrade ejaculation. Twenty-four of the patients experienced no significant changes in erectile rigidity or tumescence, while 4 had inflatable penile prostheses present prior to endoscopic ultrasonic aspiration. On long-term follow-up, no patients experienced problems with incontinence or secondary bleeding. One patient had meatal stenosis at 4 months. Two patients required transurethral incisions of the bladder neck at 12 and 15 months, respectively.

Conclusions

Ultrasonic aspiration of the prostate is being investigated to determine its proper position in the treatment of bladder outlet obstruction from benign prostatic hyperplasia. This method has proven to be an effective means of removing bladder outlet obstruction caused by prostatic adenoma. Of 40 men receiving this technique, only minimal complications were noted in patients followed for 18 months or longer.

The primary advantage of endoscopic ultrasonic aspiration of the prostate is preservation of the bladder neck, which is not cut or resected. In this limited series, the rate of retrograde ejaculation (18%) was much lower than that usually reported with electrocautery transurethral resection of the prostate. The technique can be performed effectively in a short period of time with minimal blood loss. The instrument aspirates tissue at the rate of 2 to 3 g/min. While bleeding probably averages less than with transurethral resection of the prostate, it does not constitute a major advantage of this technique. The tip of the device remains at physiologic temperatures during operation, except when electrocautery is used to control bleeding. It is felt that this helps to control any thermal injury to the periprostatic tissues, which may affect erectile function in some cases.

Any urologist skilled in transurethral resection of the prostate should be able to learn to use the ultrasonic aspirator within a short time. The cost of the procedure probably will be comparable to that of transurethral resection of the prostate, with approximately the same length of hospitalization required. It should be pointed out that proper patient selection is important, since the technique is suitable only for removing prostatic tissue and does not correct bladder neck contracture. By the same token, the bladder neck is left intact, thus minimizing retrograde ejaculation. In addition, the danger of sphincter injury also is decreased greatly.

References

1. von Ardeene M, Grossman H: Ultrasonic mechanisms for assisting in the insertion of needles in organisms. Presented at the Third International Conference

on Medical Electronics in Medicine. Institution of Electrical Engineers 1960; 3:425.

2. Kelman CD: Phaco-emulsifications and aspiration. A Report of 500 consecutive cases. *Am J Ophthalmol* 1973; 75:764–768.
3. Flamm ES, Ransohoff J, Wuchinich D, et al: Preliminary experience with ultrasonic aspiration in neurosurgery. *Neurosurgery* 1978; 2:240–245.
4. Hodgson WJ: The ultrasonic scalpel. *Bull N Y Acad Med* 1979; 55:908–915.
5. Chopp RT, Shah BB, Addonizio JC: Use of ultrasonic surgical aspirator in renal surgery. *Urology* 1983; 22:157.
6. Addonizio JC, Choudhury MS, Sayegh N, et al: Cavitron ultrasonic aspirator. *Urology* 1984; 23:417–420.
7. Addonizio JC, Choudhury MS: Cavitrons in urologic surgery. *Urol Clin North Am* 1986; 13:445–454.
8. Malloy TR, Carpiniello VL, Payne C, et al: Transurethral ultrasonic aspiration of the prostate (abstract). *J Urol* 1989; 141:342.

Balloon Dilatation of the Prostate

Lester A. Klein, M.D.

Urologist, Scripps Clinic and Research Institute, La Jolla, Californiai

This book, *Advances in Urology,* is designed to keep urologists up to date because, as practitioners of the art, we insist upon remaining current. But today, in addition to the intrinsic drive to remain abreast of the times, there are extrinsic forces upon the specialty that motivate continued learning and change. Indeed, there is a revolution in all medicine caused by (1) a trend toward nationalization of the health care system and the intervention of Congress in the daily affairs of medicine; (2) the impact of the media in distributing information to an increasingly aware and often angry public; (3) a blurring of specialty lines and the willingness, for example, of radiologists to treat obstructive prostatic disease; and (4) advances in science, which are the ideal, and perhaps should be the only, force behind change. Taken together, these factors propel new ideas, such as balloon dilatation of the prostate, onto the center stage of medicine and urology.

Balloon dilatation of the prostate is a novel and controversial approach to the care of obstructive prostatism. Clearly, it is a counterintuitive modality, because it challenges the fundamental concept of most urologists that the cause of prostatism is enlargement of the prostate gland which, by virtue of its bulk, blocks the flow of urine. Thus, when first presented with the idea, urologists tend to be skeptical of its efficacy. But empirical studies from many centers, as reviewed in this chapter, indicate that it is indeed efficacious.

On its own merit, balloon dilatation would not arouse much interest, or at least would not have aroused the interest it has so quickly, were it not for the revolution in medicine I have described. Congress wants costs cut (balloon dilatation is cheaper than prostatectomy), the public wants safe and less invasive procedures (balloon dilatation causes fewer problems than prostatectomy and requires a briefer recovery time), and interventional radiologists are willing to treat prostatism with balloons; therefore, urologists, quick to note their special background and interest in prostatic disease, have tempered their skepticism of balloon dilatation enough to take an honest, objective, scientific look at it.

Reprinted from *Advances in Urology,*® vol. 4.
Copyright 1991, Mosby–Year Book, Inc.

History

Balloon angioplasty began in the 1960s and by the beginning of the 1980s its success was widely known. The analogy between dilatation of blood vessels and dilatation of the prostatic urethra appealed to the radiologist Burhenne and his coworkers[1] who, under fluoroscopy, dilated the prostatic urethras of ten cadavers. Autopsy revealed no significant damage to the prostatic or membranous urethra and, having shown that, Burhenne became the first doctor to perform balloon dilatation of the prostate; simultaneously, he became the first patient to have his prostate dilated by balloon!

Castañeda and colleagues[2] studied the effect of balloon dilatation of the canine prostate. Under general anesthesia, a retrograde urethrogram was made to define and mark the location of the external sphincter, even though, as the authors note, this is not the optimal modality for evaluating the prostatic urethra. In a series of 28 dogs, they examined variables such as inflation pressure, balloon diameter, and duration of dilatation, and established methodological parameters that are the basis for all dilatation methods in use today. They observed that the pressure in the balloon tended to decrease during dilatation and concluded that the compliance of the prostate and its capsule were responsible for the drift. Most importantly, they showed minimal damage to the prostate and surrounding tissues and therefore suggested that dilatations in humans likely would be safe.

Castañeda and coworkers[3] then reported the results of dilatation in five patients who volunteered to undergo the procedure. Balloon dilatation was performed under fluoroscopic guidance using steerable guidewires to position the catheter. The sphincter was identified on a preliminary retrograde urethrogram and subsequently located by placing a corresponding radiopaque needle in the sheets. Further, the balloon was palpated per rectum once it was inflated. Dilatation to 75 F was done under topical anesthesia supplemented by intravenous sedation. There was radiological and clinical improvement in four of the five patients. The one who failed to improve had cystoscopic evidence of middle lobe hypertrophy, which had been shown earlier not to respond to dilatation performed with a metal dilator.[4] Magnetic resonance imaging studies of these five patients showed no evidence of intraprostatic or periprostatic hematoma.

Independently and without knowledge of the work of Burhenne and Castañeda, Dr. Brian Leeming and I began a clinical investigation of balloon dilatation in Boston in 1985. We observed the results in five patients over a 3-year period before publishing them in 1989.[5] A 36-F, 4 cm–long balloon was inflated to 5 atm in the prostatic urethra under fluoroscopic guidance for 30 minutes using local anesthesia and systemic sedation. Eight patients were prepared for dilatation, five were selected at random to undergo the procedure, and three served as controls. Two of the five patients improved clinically and urodynamically for the full 3-year follow-up period, while none of the control patients improved at all.

Development of Transcystoscopic Balloon Dilatation

The Boston study demonstrated three important factors:

1. Balloon dilatation is effective even under adverse conditions (i.e., no attempt to select ideal patients; balloons designed for angioplasty, not urethroplasty; and localization limited by the capability of fluoroscopy). It was concluded that a balloon designed specifically for prostate dilatation probably would improve the results greatly.

2. Dilatation balloons have a strong tendency to migrate and it is necessary to pull on the catheter for the duration of the procedure with a force of 45 to 75 lb. Clearly, the ideal system would obviate the need for the application of such force by overcoming migration.

3. Working with a radiologist creates scheduling problems and ultimately will lead to unnecessarily high costs. The ideal system would be one managed solely by a urologist using familiar instruments. These considerations led to the development of the transcystoscopic balloon dilata-

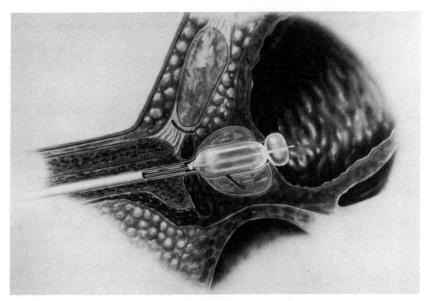

FIG. 1.
The drawing shows the essential features of the TCU catheter in relation to the anatomic structures of the lower urinary tract. The dilatation balloon is noted to completely fill the prostatic fossa yet not extend into the bladder nor the distal urethra. The placement balloon, within the bladder lumen, marks the location of the bladder neck and serves as a guide in the positioning of the dilatation balloon. The white band, noted in the drawing to be at the external sphincter, is viewed through the cytoscope during the dilatation procedure; its constancy ensures that migration of the system has not occurred.

KCOM Dept. of Surgery

tion system. Concurrently, two other nonfluoroscopic methodologies were developed. All three are described as follows.

The transcystoscopic balloon dilatation method was presented to the American Urological Association in May 1989 and was published recently in detail.[6] The dilatation balloon is passed into the bladder through a cystoscope. It is withdrawn slowly until a marker band becomes visible just distal to the external sphincter. Positioning of this band is made easy by the inflation of a Foley balloon just at the bladder side of the bladder neck (Fig 1). Under direct vision, the dilatation balloon is inflated and its proper position guaranteed by direct observation. It is not necessary to use fluoroscopy or transrectal palpation to localize the balloon. Furthermore, because of features described as follows, there is no tendency for this balloon to migrate into the bladder and therefore no traction or traction-preventing device is needed. This system, called TCU (transcystoscopic urethroplasty) and marketed by Advanced Surgical Intervention has been approved for distribution by the U.S. Food and Drug Administration since early 1988.

Other Nonfluoroscopic Balloon Dilatation Systems

A balloon dilatation system developed in collaboration with Dr. Joseph Dowd utilizes a positioning nodule or button that can be felt by digital examination via the rectum.[7] The 19-F button is positioned on the 12-F polyethylene catheter about 1 cm proximal to the dilatation balloon. A 0.038-in. guidewire is passed through a cystoscope into the bladder, the cystoscope is removed, and the dilatation catheter is passed over the guidewire. The position of the prostatic apex is determined by digital palpation and the catheter is withdrawn slowly from the bladder until the positioning nodule is felt at the apex. An assistant inflates the balloon while the operator palpates the positioning nodule, thus ensuring its position. In addition, the operator holds traction on a collar located at the distal end of the catheter in order to prevent migration of the balloon out of the prostatic urethra and into the bladder. This system, called the Dowd catheter and marketed by Microvasive, has been approved for distribution by the U.S. Food and Drug Administration.

A third nonfluoroscopic balloon dilatation system utilizes a fixation balloon that is inflated within the bulbous urethra where it can be palpated during the dilatation process. This system, presented by Reddy, Wasserman, and Sidi[8] employs a 14-F catheter that is passed into the bladder over a 0.038-in. guidewire. Initially, both balloons are passed into the lumen of the bladder. With a finger in the rectum, the apex of the prostate is palpated. The fixation balloon is inflated partially and the catheter withdrawn gently until the rectal finger palpates this balloon. Then the catheter is withdrawn a further 1.5 cm and the base of the dilating balloon may be felt. The fixation balloon will be in the urethra, just distal to the sphincter and the dilating balloon in the prostatic urethra. The fixation balloon is inflated to 40 F. As the dilatation balloon is inflated, the fixation balloon prevents it from migrating into the bladder by abutting against the sphincter. This system, called the Optilume and marketed by American Medical Systems, has been approved for distribution by the U.S. Food and Drug Administration.

Physiology of Balloon Dilatation

There is no change in the mass of adenomatous tissue following balloon dilatation documented by either ultrasound or digital rectal examination. In cases in which transurethral prostatectomy has followed balloon dilatation and in a series of needle biopsies following dilatation,[9] there has been no evidence of ischemic change of the adenoma. Clearly, the mechanism of action of dilatation is not alteration of the glandular tissue. Alterations in the number[10] and function[11] of the sensory and motor nerves surrounding the capsule have been documented in the presence of benign prostatic hypertrophy. It has been suggested that the pressure of the dilatation balloon alters these nerves, but there is no direct proof of such an effect.

The most likely mechanism by which balloon dilatation relieves obstructive prostatism is stretch of the prostatic capsule. This mechanism actually was suggested first by Diesting,[4] who proposed that prolonged dilatation produced exhaustion of the elasticity of the prostatic capsule. The effect of dilatation upon the capsular fibers can be seen dramatically in a radical prostatectomy specimen subjected to in vitro balloon dilatation. There, the stretching and disruption of the connective tissue fibers are readily apparent. The capsule is composed of collagenous and elastic connective tissue and circular rings of smooth muscle in varying proportions,[12] although in a recent abstract it was suggested that the capsule is made up of a band of concentrically placed fibromuscular tissue.[13] The effect of dilatation will be long-lasting, because elastic stretch of collagenous tissue is possible only to a limited degree, beyond which stretch produces plastic deformation or tearing of fibers so the tissue will not "spring" back into shape following distention. Because the capsule is thought to be the cause of the closure pressure along the course of the urethra (i.e., the involuntary urethral sphincter), stretch of the capsule would be expected to relieve the pressures of resistance upon the urethral channel within the prostate.

The role of the capsule in the pathogenesis of obstructive voiding has been alluded to indirectly by Schafer, who refers to compressive and constrictive obstructions in the genesis of passive and dynamic urethral resistance.[14] Compressive obstruction generally is located in the proximal urethra and is caused by prostatic enlargement that creates a need for elevated pressure to allow the passage of fluid, thus limiting flow rate by excessive demand for pressure. Constrictive obstruction is characterized by a rather rigid, small cross-sectional area that limits flow rate by lumen size even at normal opening pressure. Typically, it is represented by a stricture located in the distal urethra, but the rather rigid capsule encompassing the prostatic urethra may be thought of as a unique type of constrictive obstruction also. A discussion of the mathematical and computer-assisted analysis of passive and dynamic urethral resistance is beyond the scope of this chapter, but Schafer does conclude that the effect of benign prostatic hypertrophy on urethral flow is a combined compressive and constrictive obstruction. It seems probable that the effect of transurethral prostatectomy is upon the compressive component and that dilatation works more upon the constrictive component.

The compressive-constrictive model anticipates the applications of transurethral prostatectomy and balloon dilatation clinically. It might be predicted that patients suffering mostly from the compressive effect of benign prostatic hypertrophy will do well with transurethral prostatectomy while those with dominantly constrictive obstruction will benefit from dilatation. Unfortunately, a clinical method for distinguishing the two types of obstruction may not be available yet. For example, patients with significant prostatic enlargement may have minor degrees of prostatic obstruction and those with minimal prostatic enlargement may have severe degrees of obstruction.[15] Thus, as will be seen in the section defining patient selection, prostatic size alone is not a sufficient criterion for selecting the treatment of choice.

The observation that middle-lobe hypertrophy fails to respond to balloon dilatation may be explained by the fact that the middle lobe is not enclosed within the prostatic capsule. Therefore, to the extent that the middle lobe is producing symptoms, capsular stretch will be ineffective. To the extent that an individual's symptoms are due to prostate trapped by the capsule, capsular stretch will be effective. Similarly, the bladder neck, which is not enclosed by capsule, will not be altered effectively by balloon dilatation.

Ideally, the capsule should be stretched in its entirety, that is, from apex to bladder neck. Unlike transurethral prostatectomy, dilatation must go distal to the verumontanum; fortunately, this does not result in any degree of incontinence. The design of the balloon is critical in achieving this goal. The best angle of the shoulders that connect the balloon to the catheter shaft has been found by empirical and anatomical studies to be 60 degrees.[6] Steeper shoulders may injure the apical area. Any tendency of the balloon to migrate cephalad into the bladder will make it difficult to realize dilatation of the apical area and that may reduce the ultimate effectiveness of the dilatation. The diameter of the balloon is important also. While it would seem that "bigger is better," that is not the case, because applying a big balloon to a small gland could severely rupture the gland. Thus, 75 F seems a safe compromise, since it will not injure a small gland, and larger glands (>40 g) should be subjected to prostatectomy.

Preoperative Evaluation of the Patient

The most important feature of the balloon dilatation candidate is that he be symptomatic. One of the most significant and useful advances in the practice of urology is the objective symptom score analysis form developed in Madison, Wisconsin.[16] It is an excellent tool for both the initial and follow-up evaluations of patients with benign prostatic hypertrophy, whether they are treated or not, dilated or resected. Most current outcome reports utilize this analytical tool. It distinguishes irritative from obstructive symptoms and is weighted toward the latter. The test is either self-administered or given by a health technician. In follow-up, the patient does not see his earlier responses. The minimal score that should arouse interest in interventional therapy is 9 or 10. A urodynamic evaluation is recommended, although the urodynamic parameter that should be measured is unclear. We have found the uroflow, especially the peak uroflow, to be the most reliable, easily obtainable parameter. Peak uroflow under 10 mL/sec should arouse suspicion of obstruction, and flows below 5 ml/sec may indicate advanced obstruction or bladder decompensation. The best candidates seem to have peak flows between 5 and 10 mL/sec. Urinary tract infection and prostatitis should be ruled out. Because no tissue is obtained with dilatation, in contrast to transurethral prostatectomy, the discovery of occult or small carcinomas will be missed. In order to mitigate that possibility, every patient who is to be dilated must be screened with prostate-specific antigen and transrectal ultrasound. Although these steps probably will not discover as many occult neoplasms as will prostatectomy, it is this author's view that many of the patients who are candidates for balloon dilatation would not be candidates for prostatectomy and therefore would not be subjected to histological evaluation of their prostates in any case. Further, since the group of dilated patients tends to be younger than the prostatectomy group, there is a lesser incidence of prostatic cancer. Finally, patients should have cystoscopy to rule out incidental lower urinary tract pathology and to evaluate the condition of the middle lobe. The flexible cystoscope is superior to the rigid cystoscope in the evaluation of the middle lobe.

Balloon Dilatation and Urodynamics

Dilating the urinary passageway for the relief of prostatism is based on the idea that outflow obstruction produces symptoms and elimination of obstruction produces relief. Logically, it follows that a successful dilatation would yield objective improvement in urinary flow. Although such improvement has been recorded, the correlation between symptomatic and urodynamic improvement following balloon dilatation is not strong.[17] The absence of a correlation between symptomatic and urodynamic outcome is not unique; a similarly poor correlation has been found in the outcome of prostatectomy.[18, 19] An explanation for this discrepancy is elusive,[20] and even bladder instability, which is commonly thought to be responsible for the failure of many transurethral resections,[21] does not correlate well with the clinical outcome of prostatectomy.[18]

In attempting to reconcile the difference between symptomatic and urodynamic improvement following the treatment of prostatism, it must be recognized that over 90% of prostatectomies are performed for symptoms, not for abnormal urodynamic findings.[22] Therefore, it has been suggested that a clinical analysis of symptoms is a better predictor of the outcome of prostatectomy than are urodynamic findings.[23] Despite predictions that more sophisticated urodynamic parameters (e.g., the micturition index[24]) would improve the postprostatectomy correlation of symptoms with urodynamics,[25] this has not occurred, and today, the best yardstick for a successful prostatectomy is the improvement the patient experiences in quality of life. What is true for prostatectomy is also true for balloon dilatation: the most consistent measure of success is symptom analysis, not "objective" urodynamic parameters.[26] The symptom score sheet[16] is an excellent tool for postoperative evaluation of the patient. A successful response to balloon dilatation is defined as a drop in symptoms of at least 50%, although patients with a 33% reduction in symptoms are satisfied.[26]

Review of the Literature

To date, very little has appeared in the peer-reviewed literature regarding balloon dilatation of the prostate. Primarily, abstracts have been published in connection with meetings such as that of the American Urological Association. Dowd and Smith reported 58% improvement in patients, 30% of whom had been in refractory retention, 61% of whom had failed a trial of α-blockers, and 42% of whom were too ill to be subjected to transurethral prostatectomy.[27] Immediate improvement has been reported in 70% to 80% of patients, but their relapse rates were reported at 3% and 70%.[28, 29] The variance between 3% and 70% may be understood in light of two important variables: the method of balloon dilatation and the patient selection process. The group reporting a 70% relapse rate used a fluoroscopic method of dilatation and did not choose patients now known to be more appropriate candidates (at the time, patient stratification was not clear.)

A careful analysis of a report[30] in which only 11% of patients improved with balloon dilatation reveals two features that might explain the low success rate: (1) a figure of an x-ray demonstrates that the dilatation balloon appears to be inflated primarily within the bladder and not the prostatic urethra, thus mitigating its effect on the prostatic capsule; and (2) the average prostate size was 69 g, which is much larger than the maximum size successfully dilated in other studies where glands over 40 g usually failed to respond to dilatation.[17, 26] Parenthetically, if in fact the dilatation was not technically effective, then it may be suggested that the reported improvement rate of 11% represents the placebo effect rate for balloon dilatation. The value of 11% is substantially less than the placebo rate for medications taken for prostatism.[31] Perhaps the explanation for medication being a more effective placebo is that it is taken over a long period of time, reinforcing its presence, whereas the effect of dilatation, as a single-episode intervention, may dwindle in significance over time.

In our own work, we have followed 22 patients for over 24 months and another 44 for 1 to 16 months. Among the initial 22 patients, 7 failed within the first 6 months after dilatation and another 3 did so within the next 6 months. One failed between the first and second year. Thus, 10 of 11 failures occurred within 1 year. In retrospect, those 10 patients had either prostate glands >40 g, flow rates <5 mL/sec, large middle lobes, or prostatitis. Had they not been dilated, the success rate at 2 years would have been 11 of 12. That is borne out by the results of the next 44 patients, among whom the success rate was 93%, and who had none of the aforementioned conditions.[32]

An Algorithm for Selecting Treatment for Patients with Benign Prostatic Hypertrophy

In analyzing our results, several parameters emerge that are associated with failure. Patients with middle-lobe hypertrophy, peak uroflow rates below 5 mL/sec, or glands over 40 g generally are not improved by balloon dilatation.[26] These are precisely the patients whose prostatism is best managed by prostatectomy.[33] Therefore, if the patient has a very restricted uroflow, a large gland, or a large middle lobe, prostatectomy is recommended; small glands associated with better uroflows are recommended for balloon dilatation. In practice, most patients who are candidates for balloon dilatation are given a trial of adrenergic blockers if their general medical condition permits. Those who fail medications are advanced to balloon intervention. This triage process maximizes the potential success rate and reduces the complication rate. Because there is an increased incidence of postoperative bladder neck contractures in surgery for small prostates,[34] avoiding operation of these is indicated.

Postoperative Management

With few exceptions, postoperative management after balloon dilatation is similar to that following transurethral prostatectomy. A Foley catheter is kept in place for 48 to 72 hours, not to control bleeding, but because it has been observed that some patients develop transient urinary retention after being dilated (perhaps due to swelling of the prostatic urethra). I use a double-balloon Foley catheter (such as a Coleman catheter) with the second balloon inflated to 5 to 10 mL within the prostatic fossa to achieve tamponade. The prostatic balloon is deflated within hours. Bladder spasms are controlled with either belladonna or pain medication and antibiotics may be selected. After the catheter is removed, the patient may complain of urinary frequency and urgency and perhaps experience transient dribbling and nocturia. Patients go home the day of dilatation or spend 1 night in the hospital. Rarely do patients require more attention.

Complications

The most common complication of the balloon procedure is failure of the patient to improve following dilatation. However, our experience has shown that this almost always can be attributed to poor patient selection, i.e., one with an overall gland or middle lobe that is too enlarged or a bladder that is decompensated. Three patients out of 66 (4.5%) went into total retention for over 2 weeks, at which point transurethral prostatectomy relieved them. There was no undue difficulty with the operations in that small group. One patient required transfusion; because of the presence of an artificial aortic valve, he was fully anticoagulated and control was not achieved until the anticoagulation was reversed. Among over 3,000 patients dilated with the TCU transcystoscopic system, no incontinence or retrograde ejaculation has been reported.

Role of Balloon Dilatation in Clinical Practice

Balloon dilatation is an important addition to the urologist's armamentarium. It extends our capacity to deliver care to a large group of patients who are not good candidates for transurethral prostatectomy on the grounds that they are too young or otherwise reluctant or ineligible to undergo a surgical procedure. Further, it is the ideal modality for the patient with a small but highly symptomatic prostate gland. The number of such patients may be very large. For example, in a study of 3,885 prostatectomies, 33% of the specimens were <10 g and 50% were <22 g.[22] Because balloon dilatation is less costly than prostatectomy, the savings for third-party payors is significant. The economic impact to urologists may be small or even favorable in view of the potential increase in our ability to deliver care to a large proportion of patients. Finally, the joy of practice increases when there are several therapeutic options available and we are called upon to guide our patients through the maze toward the best outcome.

References

1. Burhenne GH, Chisholm RJ, Quenville NF: Prostatic hyperplasia: Radiological intervention. Radiology 1984; 152:655–657.
2. Castañeda F, Lund G, Larson BW, et al: Prostatic urethra: Experimental dilation in dogs. Radiology 1987; 163:645–648.
3. Castañeda F, Reddy P, Wasserman N, et al: Benign prostatic hypertrophy: Retrograde transurethral dilation of the prostatic urethra in humans. Radiology 1987; 163:649–653.
4. Deisting W: Transurethral dilatation of the prostate. Urol Int 1956; 2:158–171.
5. Klein LA, Leeming B: Balloon dilatation for prostatic obstruction. Urology 1989; 33:198–201.

6. Klein L, Abrams P: Transurethral cystoscopic balloon dilatation of the prostate. *Problems in Urology* 1989; 3:395–402.
7. Dowd JB: Non-surgical treatment of benign prostatic hypertrophy. Presented at the annual meeting of the American Urological Association. Dallas, Texas, May 1989.
8. Reddy PK, Wasserman N, Sidi A: Balloon dilation of the prostate: Can it help the patient with BPH. *Contemp Urol* 1989; 144–53.
9. Benson R, personal communication, 1990.
10. Gosling JA, Gilpin SA, Dixon JS, et al: Decrease in the autonomic innervation of human detrusor muscle in outflow obstruction. *J Urol* 1986; 136:501–504.
11. Chalfin SA, Bradley WE: The etiology of detrusor hyperreflexia in patients with infravesical obstruction. *J Urol* 1982; 127:938–942.
12. Hutch JA, Rambo ON: A study of the anatomy of the prostate, prostatic urethra and the urinary sphincter system. *J Urol* 1970; 104S:443–452.
13. Alaya AG: Existence of prostatic capsule debated. *Urol Times* 1990; 18:5.
14. Schafer W: *Benign Prostatic Hypertrophy.* New York, Springer-Verlag, 1983.
15. Yalla SV, Blute B, Waters WB, et al: Urodynamic evaluation of prostatic enlargements with micturitional vesicourethral static pressure profiles. *J Urol* 1981; 125:685–689.
16. Frimodt-Moller PC, Jensen KME, Iversen P, et al: Analysis of presenting symptoms in prostatism. *J Urol* 1984; 132:272–276.
17. Goldenberg SL, Perez-Marrero RA, Lee LM, et al: Endoscopic balloon dilation of the prostate: Early experience. *J Urol* 1990; 144:83–88.
18. Abrams PH, Farrar DJ, Turner-Warwick RT, et al: The results of prostatectomy: A symptomatic and urodynamic analysis of 152 patients. *J Urol* 1979; 121:640–642.
19. Susset JG, Dutarte D: Evaluation of urinary flow rate with prostatectomy. *Urology* 1975; 5:763–768.
20. Graversen PH, Gasser TC, Wasson JH, et al: Controversies about indications for transurethral resection of the prostate. *J Urol* 1989; 141:475–481.
21. Abrams PH: Investigation of post prostatectomy problems. *Urology* 1980; 15:209–212.
22. Mebust WK, Holtgrewe HL, Cockett ATK, et al: Transurethral prostatectomy: Immediate and postoperative complications. Cooperative study of 13 participating institutions evaluating 3885 patients. *J Urol* 1989; 141:243–247.
23. Bruskewitz R, Jensen KM-E, Iverson P, et al: The relevance of minimum urethral resistance in prostatism. *J Urol* 1983; 129:769–771.
24. Anderson RU: Urodynamic patterns after acute spinal cord injury. *J Urol* 1983; 129:777–779.
25. Blaivas JG: Urodynamics: The second generation. *J Urol* 1983; 129:783.
26. Klein LA, Perez-Marrero R, Bowers GW, et al: Transurethral cystoscopic balloon dilatation of the prostate. *Endourology* 1990; 4:115–123.
27. Dowd JB, Smith JJ: Balloon dilation of the prostate without imaging: Comparison with transurethral resection of the prostate. *J Urol* 1990; 143:A375.
28. Hernandez-Graulau J, Eshighi M, Choudhury M, et al: Balloon divulsion of the prostate for treatment of BPH: 18 months follow-up: Is it really worth it? *J Urol* 1990; 4S:A374.
29. Goldenberg SL, Perez-Marrero R, Lee LM, et al: Endoscopic balloon dilatation of the prostate. *J Urol* 1990; 4S:A379.
30. Gill KP, Machan LS, Allison DJ, et al: Bladder outflow tract obstruction and urinary retention from benign prostatic hypertrophy treated by balloon dilatation. *Br J Urol* 1989; 64S:618–622.

31. Abrams PJ, Shah R, Stone R, et al: Bladder outflow obstruction treated with phenoxybenzamine. *Br J Urol* 1982; 54:527–530.
32. Klein LA: Two year follow-up of balloon dilatation of the prostate and on algorithm for future patient selection. *J Endocrinol*, in press.
33. Abrams PH: Prostatism and prostatectomy: The value of urine flow rate measurement in the preoperative assessment for operation. *J Urol* 1977; 117:70–71.
34. Bruskewitz RC, Larsen EH, Madsen PO, et al: 3-year followup of urinary symptoms after transurethral resection of the prostate. *J Urol* 1986; 136:613–615.

Indications for the Use of Drugs in the Male Reproductive System*

Carol M. Proudfit, Ph.D.

Assistant Division Director, Division of Drugs and Toxicology, American Medical Association, Chicago, Illinois

Physiology

Androgens are secreted by the testes and the adrenal cortex in males. They are responsible for developing and maintaining secondary sexual characteristics, normal reproductive function, and sexual performance ability, as well as for stimulating the growth and development of the skeleton and skeletal muscle during puberty.

Testosterone is the principal androgen secreted by the steroidogenic Leydig cells, which are located in the interstitial spaces of the testis. Men produce 2.5 to 10 mg of testosterone daily and plasma concentrations are 200 to 1,000 ng/dL. Plasma levels fluctuate in a circadian pattern in young men and are maximal in the early morning. Superimposed on this rhythm are shorter, smaller secretory peaks that follow elevated luteinizing hormone (LH) secretion within hours. These variations in plasma hormone levels demonstrate the importance of multiple blood sampling in some experimental and diagnostic situations.

In males, about one third of the 17-ketosteroids (testosterone precursors) are secreted by the adrenal cortex. However, since the biopotency and rate of conversion to testosterone are low, adrenal androgens are not as important functionally as is the smaller amount of testosterone produced by the testis. If Leydig cell function is lost or markedly impaired, the amount of testosterone produced by conversion of the adrenocortical androgens, androstenedione and dehydroepiandrosterone, is inadequate to maintain normal male function.

The anterior pituitary hormone, LH, originally called interstitial cell-stimulating hormone, stimulates steroidogenesis in the Leydig cells. Follicle-stimulating hormone (FSH) is necessary for quantitatively and qualitatively normal spermatogenesis. A negative feedback system involving the hypothalamus, the anterior pituitary, and the testis controls gonadotropic hormone secretion. Testosterone suppresses secretion of LH and, to a lesser extent, FSH. Estradiol, which is secreted by the testis and produced by the

*Adapted from *Drug Evaluations Subscription.* Chicago, American Medical Association, 1990.

Reprinted from *Advances in Urology,*® vol. 4.

peripheral conversion of testosterone and other androgens, also may participate in the negative feedback control of LH and FSH. Synthetic androgens that cannot be aromatized to estrogen (e.g., oxandrolone, mesterolone) are less effective in suppressing gonadotropins than is testosterone, which can be aromatized.

Inhibin, a glycoprotein consisting of disulfide-linked α and β subunits secreted by the Sertoli cells of the seminiferous tubules, also inhibits the release of FSH. Serum inhibin concentration increases during puberty in both sexes,[1] and this glycoprotein may play a role in development of FSH target tissues (i.e., Sertoli cells, ovarian follicles) at that time.[2]

In men, approximately 98% of circulating testosterone is bound to protein, primarily to sex hormone–binding globulin (testosterone-estradiol–binding globulin) and albumin. As with other steroid hormones, the biologically active portion is the free (dialyzable, unbound) fraction. The hepatic synthesis of sex hormone–binding globulin is decreased by androgens and elevated by estrogens. Consequently, men have higher levels of free-circulating testosterone than do women, both proportionately and in total amount. In contrast, because of their high total estradiol secretion, women have higher free estradiol concentrations, even though a smaller fraction of plasma estradiol is unbound.

The half-life of endogenous free testosterone in the blood is 10 to 20 minutes. Testosterone is metabolized primarily in the liver and is excreted mainly in the urine as the metabolites androsterone and etiocholanolone. Small amounts of testosterone glucuronide and sulfate also are excreted. About 6% of the hormone is excreted unaltered in the feces. Synthetic androgens are metabolized also by reduction of the Δ 4-3 keto function and oxidation elsewhere on the molecule, but their plasma half-lives are longer because they are metabolized more slowly. Synthetic androgens may be excreted as unaltered hormone or as metabolites.

The steroidogenic activity of LH is mediated through stimulation of cyclic adenosine monophosphate (cAMP) and calmodulin synthesis. The androgenic action of testosterone in some tissues (e.g., prostate, seminal vesicle, external genitalia) normally depends upon the intracellular reduction of testosterone to 5α-dihydrotestosterone (DHT), which binds to the specific androgen receptor in the cytoplasm of these tissues. In other tissues (e.g., skeletal muscle, bone marrow, Sertoli cells), testosterone itself is probably the active intracellular hormone. In the central nervous system, the hormonal effects of testosterone may result in part from its aromatization to estradiol. The ultimate effect of the steroid-receptor complex is to influence production of messenger RNA to direct protein synthesis in the cell.

Aging

Increasing age in men has been correlated with a decreased number of Leydig cells, reduced sperm production, and elevated serum concentrations of LH and FSH. Elevation of FSH is greater and correlates with lowest sperm production.[3] In one study, testosterone not bound to sex hormone–binding globulin (albumin-bound and free testosterone) was decreased in normal older men (aged 65 to 83 years), but not in younger men (aged 22 to 39 years).[4] In other studies, free plasma testosterone was reported to decline with advancing age, which correlates with reduction of various aspects of sexuality such as frequency of activity, erectile and orgasmic function, and libido. Hormonal changes are thought to be responsible for only a small part of declining sexual activity with age.[5]

There is no male hormonal climacteric analogous to that in women. However, when serum testosterone levels decrease abruptly at any age (e.g., following surgical trauma or orchiectomy), vasomotor flushing can occur. This may be alleviated by testosterone replacement therapy.

Behavior

Because of complex and interacting variables involved in the determination of human behavior, it is not surprising that clinical studies have failed to describe consistent hormonal profiles for certain behavioral patterns in men, such as homosexuality and aggressive behavior. Data from different studies are difficult to compare because procedures have not been standardized (e.g., measurement of total vs. free testosterone, sampling at different amplitudes of the circadian cycle, lack of information on the ratio of free estrogen:testosterone). Furthermore, reported differences in hormone level may be a cause, an effect, or unrelated to behavior.

Based on results obtained in animals, behavior may be influenced by hormonal imprinting at a critical stage in development rather than by hormones present later. In some animals, for example, androgens program the brain in fetal or neonatal life and set patterns of gonadotropic hormone secretion and sexual behavior. It has been suggested that similar influences are operative in humans.[6] Psychosexual orientation that may have been influenced by prenatal hormone exposure has been described (e.g., some females with virilizing congenital adrenal hyperplasia, genetic males with 5α-reductase deficiency), but not proved.[7]

The possibility that identifiable patterns of serum hormone concentrations might serve as markers for sexual orientation is a controversial concept. Two widely quoted studies illustrate the conflicting evidence. In one study, men with lifelong homosexual orientation demonstrated a serum LH response to estrogen administration that was intermediate between that of women and that of heterosexual men; the group observation could not be extrapolated to individuals, however.[8] In a later study, no significant difference in LH response to estrogen was detected among heterosexual men, homosexual men, and transsexual women.[9]

Indications

Constitutional Delay of Growth

This condition occurs in approximately 2.5% of normal children and more frequently causes concern in boys than in girls. Family history may reveal similar growth retardation in parents, siblings, or other relatives. The diagnosis is made by exclusion and is conclusive after normal but late and prolonged pubescent development. Boys with idiopathic delayed puberty have been differentiated from those with permanent hypothalamic hypogonadism on the basis of nocturnal LH secretory patterns. Patients with delayed puberty had elevated, pulsatile patterns of nocturnal LH secretion, while those with hypothalamic hypogonadism did not. There were no differences in baseline testosterone levels or LH response to gonadotropin releasing hormone (Gn-RH) injection.[10]

Medical attention is frequently sought because of short stature rather than lack of sexual development, in contrast to patients with primary or hypogonadotropic hypogonadism, whose height is often normal but who lack sexual development. Characteristics of constitutional delayed growth include normal birth weight, growth curve parallel to normal, low bone age for chronological age but normal for the stage of development (bone age is normal in genetic short stature), and low levels of plasma gonadotropins and adrenal androgens for age but normal for size and stage of sexual development.[11-13]

Bone age is determined at the initial evaluation. Family history of growth development is obtained and nonendocrine causes of growth retardation are considered. Further testing may be postponed during a 6-month observation period unless the child is three or more standard deviations below average height or there is no sexual maturation by the bone age of 12 to 13 years or the chronological age of 14 years in boys. Extreme anxiety of the patient and parents also may stimulate earlier evaluation. Serum thyroxine and gonadotropins are measured and, if normal, the adequacy of growth hormone secretion may be determined.

Treatment.—Drug therapy is not required to achieve normal growth in constitutional delay of growth and puberty; normal development occurs by 18 years and full adult height is usually within the normal range, although linear growth may not be complete until after 20 years of age. However, when delayed growth and puberty cause significant emotional stress despite reassurance, treatment with androgenic agents may be considered in boys.

The goal of therapy is to accelerate initiation of a growth spurt that otherwise would occur later. Patients should be 14 years or older with a bone age at least 2 years behind the chronological age before treatment is attempted. Care must be taken to avoid doses that produce premature epiphyseal closure, which would compromise adult height. Usually, hormone treatment is employed for 3 to 6 months, followed by a drug-free observation period of 6 months. Bone age should be determined roentgenographically before the initiation of therapy and at intervals during and after treatment. The increase in bone age should not exceed the increase in height age. Since stimulation of bone maturation may persist for 6 months after therapy is discontinued, steroids should be withdrawn well before the skeletal age reaches the norm for the chronological age. Often the pubertal changes initiated by treatment proceed spontaneously after one course of therapy, but a second course may be employed if necessary. However, the need for a second course should prompt reconsideration of the diagnosis of gonadotropin deficiency.

Any anabolic steroid or androgen may be prescribed for constitutional delay of growth. The choice of preparation depends on the balance of growth stimulation and sexual maturation desired. The route of administration preferred also may influence drug selection. Oxandrolone (Anavar), an oral anabolic steroid, has been used for this purpose in the past, but it is no longer marketed. A preparation with greater androgenic activity, usually an intramuscular testosterone ester (e.g., testosterone enanthate [Andryl, Delatestryl]), may be chosen if stimulation of sexual development is desired and growth potential has been achieved or nearly so.

Cryptorchidism

Little spontaneous testicular descent occurs after 12 months of age, and progressive irreversible tubular damage may begin in cryptorchid testes by the first or second year of life; therefore, treatment should begin early to avoid infertility. Initiation of drug therapy is usually recommended by 2 years of age. However, some tubular function may be preserved even when treatment is started in prepubertal boys; delay until puberty usually results in the inability to produce sperm. Even after testicular descent, normal spermatogenesis may not occur. Among men who underwent orchiopexy for cryptorchidism, the paternity rate was higher in those with unilateral than bilateral cryptorchidism.[14] Androgen production is rarely compromised in the cryptorchid testis.

Men with a history of cryptorchidism have an increased relative risk of developing testicular cancer. Although the estimates vary greatly, a relative risk 8 times higher than normal for bilateral cryptorchidism and 6.5 times higher than normal for unilateral cryptorchidism seems likely.[15] Formerly, it was thought that the relative risk of testicular cancer was as high as 35, but the lower estimates cited now appear to be more realistic. A relative risk of testicular cancer, 5.9 times higher than that in noncryptorchid subjects was found in another study. In unilateral cryptorchidism, the risk of cancer was higher in the affected testis.[16] About 10% of men with testicular cancer have a history of cryptorchidism.[17] Although questions remain about the relationship between correlation of cryptorchidism and testicular cancer,[15, 18] a case-control study on 271 patients with testicular cancer provided the first direct, although limited, evidence that the risk increases with age at correction.[19] Even though correction of cryptorchidism does not always prevent malignancy, it facilitates detection if malignancy does occur.

Treatment.—Correction of cryptorchidism at an early age currently is recommended to preserve fertility and prevent testicular cancer. Because of its safety and the possibility of success, hormonal therapy probably should be employed before surgery is undertaken. If this is unsuccessful, surgical correction (or removal of the cryptorchid testis if this fails) should be performed.

Chorionic gonadotropin (CG) has been the standard hormonal therapy for this condition. Gonadorelin (Gn-RH) also shows promise as a therapeutic agent in properly selected subjects. Success rates for hormonal therapy of cryptorchid testes vary widely. Discrepancies may be due to failure to differentiate between retractile and true cryptorchid testes. In a double-blind study in which 33 patients with retractile testes were excluded, neither subcutaneously administered hCG nor intranasally administered gonadorelin stimulated testicular descent; in 5 boys with retractile testes, hCG induced testicular descent.[20] In a double-blind placebo-controlled study of 252 cryptorchid boys, treatment with gonadorelin nasal spray caused testicular descent in only 18% of subjects. Moreover, the clinical description of the successfully treated subjects suggests that about half had retractile and not truly cryptorchid testes.[21, 22]

Hypogonadism

Decreased Leydig cell function can result from abnormality of the testis (primary hypogonadism) or from lack of gonadotropic stimulation (hypogonadotropism) caused by hypothalamic (tertiary) or pituitary (secondary) failure. In one study, almost all patients with idiopathic hypogonadotropic hypogonadism lacked pulsatile LH or FSH secretion. The most severely affected patients had never undergone puberty, and half of these also were anosmic. Other patients in whom pulsatile gonadotropin secretion was lacking experienced at least partial spontaneous puberty. Other aberrations in the patterns of gonadotropic secretion include nocturnal pulses similar to those in early puberty and low-amplitude gonadotropin pulses.[23]

Disorders associated with primary Leydig cell failure include chromosomal defect (e.g., Klinefelter's syndrome), trauma, irradiation, or testicular failure associated with disease (e.g., myotonic dystrophy, mumps orchitis). Serum gonadotropin levels are high in primary failure (due to lack of negative feedback by androgen) and low in secondary hypogonadism. Patients with primary or secondary hypogonadism may seek help because of failure of normal pubertal development or because of impotence, lack of libido, infertility, or decreased beard growth after pubertal development was completed.

Testicular response to gonadotropin may be tested by administering hCG. If testosterone secretion is stimulated markedly, primary gonadal failure or insensitivity to gonadotropin is ruled out. hCG also can be used to stimulate testicular function, but treatment is inconvenient and expensive and generally is not used except for infertility.

The time to initiate replacement therapy depends on when clinical manifestations appear, not on whether hypogonadism is primary or secondary. For example, patients with primary testicular failure may not seek medical attention until adulthood. A patient with Klinefelter's syndrome may have normal height, incomplete virilization, and eunuchoid body proportions but may not consult a physician until infertility becomes apparent in adulthood.

Treatment.—Regardless of the cause of hypogonadism, the dose and schedule for replacement therapy depend on age and development stage at presentation and the severity of the deficit. Therapy may be directed toward induction of puberty, maintenance of secondary sexual characteristics and sexual behavior, or treatment of infertility. When *induction of puberty* is undertaken, a parenteral preparation such as testosterone enanthate or testosterone cypionate (Andro-Cyp, Depo-Testosterone) achieves best results. Replacement dosages are generally increased to induce progressive changes of puberty, and full sexual development is usually attained in 3 to 4 years. Priapism, which is rarely a problem with appropriate dosage, can be alleviated by adjusting the amount given. Although oral therapy with fluoxymesterone (Halotestin) or methyltestosterone (Metandren, Oreton Methyl, Testred) may be more convenient for maintenance therapy in patients with hypogonadism, the parenteral testosterone esters are preferred for long-term use because of their greater potency and avoidance of the hepatotoxicity associated with 17 α-alkylated compounds.

An investigational transdermal system consisting of a self-adhering film impregnated with testosterone has been successful in providing testosterone in a pattern that mimics normal circadian secretion. A patch is applied daily to the scrotal skin, which is highly permeable because of its vascularity and thin stratum corneum.[24] Normal serum testosterone concentrations, as well as satisfactory secondary sexual characteristics, libido, and sexual function, are achieved. However, greatly increased levels of DHT are found, probably due to 5α-reductase activity and conversion from testosterone in the scrotal skin. More studies are necessary to determine if long-term risks such as prostatic hypertrophy are associated with the elevated DHT levels.[25–27]

Impotence

Erection involves complex interactions of psychological, hormonal, neural, and vascular functions. Both sympathetic and parasympathetic pathways are utilized. In the flaccid state, α-1-postjunctional adrenoreceptor stimulation of smooth tone in arterioles probably maintains restricted blood flow. Relaxation of smooth muscle in arterioles and sinusoids of the corpora cavernosa and spongiosum reduces peripheral resistance and increases blood flow and engorgement of these tissues. Although acetylcholine may initiate this relaxation, vasoactive intestinal polypeptide may be one of the major neurotransmitters to produce this effect. Compression of venules, probably a passive phenomenon, helps maintain the erection.[28, 29]

Impotence may result from malfunction of one or more of the functional support systems. In the past, it was thought the impotence was of psychogenic origin in more than 90% of the cases. Although there is frequently a psychologic component, organic causes are identified now in about 50% of the cases. Neurologic causes include impotence secondary to a disease (e.g., diabetes mellitus, multiple sclerosis) and spinal cord injury or nerve damage caused by surgery (e.g., prostatectomy). Decreased blood flow to the penis due to factors such as arteriosclerosis, vascular damage from injury, bypass procedure, or renal transplantation; endocrine malfunction from conditions including hypogonadism and hyperprolactinemia; or structural abnormality of the penis caused by deviations such as Peyronie's disease also may cause impotence. Numerous drugs can induce erectile dysfunction also including most antihypertensive agents, opioids, antidepressants, antianxiety and antipsychotic agents, ethyl alcohol, chemotherapeutic agents, cimetidine, and estrogenic agents).[30-32] Reviews on impotence in diabetes[33] and in the elderly[34] are available.

Diagnosis.—Initial diagnostic efforts are directed toward determining whether impotence is psychogenic or organic. A complete physical examination is performed and a history is taken; the latter includes sexual history and questioning about recent emotional upheavals or use of drugs that could affect erectile function. Psychogenic impotence is more likely to be abrupt in onset and of a situational nature (e.g., to vary in occurrence or severity with different partners or techniques). Organic impotence tends to be gradual in onset and occurs more consistently.

Assessment of nocturnal penile tumescence can help differentiate psychogenic from organic impotence. Normal men experience one to several erections during nighttime sleep. Men with psychogenic impotence continue to have erections during sleep but are unable to experience or maintain an erection while awake. Several mechanical and electronic devices are available to measure nocturnal penile tumescence. The former type consists of a band placed around the base of the penis. The band is calibrated so that closure made of velcro or plastic break at various levels of pressure.[35] Further refinement of nocturnal penile tumescence assessment has taken into account changes in both circumference and rigidity; the latter is determined by the use of microprocessors, servomotors, and loop transducers. A simple but crude mechanical method of nocturnal penile tumescence assessment is to secure a strip of stamps around the base of the penis; if erection occurs during the night, the strip is broken.[36]

Intracavernous injection of papaverine also has been used as a screening technique. Patients who fail to have an erection following this procedure probably have vasogenic impotence; patients who respond positively may be spared angiography.[37, 38] Other diagnostic methods are used to investigate neural (e.g., evoked potentials in the pudendal nerve) and vascular (e.g., angiography, Doppler pulse-wave analysis) causes of impotence. Diagnostic methods for vascular,[39] neural,[40] and hormonal[41] causes of impotence have been reviewed.

Treatment.—The method of treatment for impotence depends on the cause. Psychogenic impotence often can be treated successfully in sex therapy programs, but this approach can be lengthy. Vascular causes may be correctable by surgery to repair damaged arteries or tie off leaky veins. Penile prosthetic implants, available as semirigid, inflatable, or articulating devices,[42] are effective for impotence from any cause, but should be used only when other methods are unsuitable or fail. A penile implant may preclude the occurrence of a natural erection. A discussion of therapeutic options for the treatment of impotence is available.[43]

Pharmacologic treatment also is sometimes appropriate. In hypogonadal men, testosterone replacement can restore libido and potency. The effectiveness of androgen therapy in the absence of low serum testosterone is unproven. Some patients helped by empiric therapy may have an underlying gonadal disorder (for instance, some diabetic patients have gonadal dysfunction due to diabetes).[44] The possibility of stimulating prostate growth in older men should be considered before prescribing testosterone without a clear need for replacement.[45] Hyperprolactinemia in men is often accompanied by low serum testosterone and impotence. Bromocriptine lowers or normalizes the serum prolactin concentration, and this is often accompanied by a return of potency (see the discussion on infertility due to hyperprolactinemia). In these instances, administration of testosterone alone generally is ineffective.[29] Patients with hyperprolactinemia and impotence should be evaluated for pituitary tumor prior to initiating therapy with bromocriptine.

Yohimbine has long been reputed to be an aphrodisiac. Determination of its effectiveness for the treatment of impotence has been impeded by experimental designs that utilized combination regimens and had other deficiencies. In the study most often cited to date, 23 patients with organic impotence not associated with hypothalamic-pituitary-gonadal deficiency were given yohimbine (Yohimex) 6 mg orally three times daily for 10 weeks. This uncontrolled study showed improved quality or complete return of erectile function in 17% and 26% of subjects, respectively (43% positive response).[46] Minor side effects, which included nausea, nervousness, and/or dizziness, were reported by 3 patients. Larger doses caused weakness, elevated blood pressure, and increased heart rate. In later controlled studies by the same group, subjects with organic impotence received the same regimen as previously stated; the response rate for yohimbine was 43.5% vs. 27.6% for those who received a placebo, a difference that was not statistically significant.[47] In another study in men with psychogenic impotence, the effect of yohimbine was statistically significant compared with that of placebo.[48]

Yohimbine is an α_2-adrenergic antagonist. It purportedly affects erectile function by enhancing norepinephrine release; this blocks the presynaptic alpha receptor and causes either increased arterial inflow or reduced venous outflow.[49] Yohimbine may stimulate erotically induced erection via a sympathetic pathway rather than reflex erection via a parasympathetic pathway, as evidenced by failure to produce nocturnal penile tumescence.[50] At this time, documentation of yohimbine's usefulness to treat impotence is sparse and inconclusive. Although the drug may be useful in some patients and is probably worthy of further investigation, its use for the treatment of impotence remains unproven.

The most widely used new pharmacologic treatment for impotence is the injection of papaverine[51] or, more commonly, papaverine plus phentolamine, into the corpus cavernosum. Papaverine is a smooth muscle relaxant and phentolamine is an α-adrenergic blocking agent. Together, these agents increase blood flow by promoting smooth muscle relaxation in penile arterioles and sinusoids. In addition, papaverine has been reported to increase venous resistance. Although papaverine can stimulate an erection when given alone, the addition of phentolamine potentiates the effect.[28]

In uncontrolled trials employing intracorporal injections of papaverine and phentolamine, 16 of 21 patients reported a positive response[52]; another study of 100 men with organic impotence reported a 100% response in patients with neurogenic impotence, a 90% response in patients with impotence of undetermined cause, and a 66% response in patients with vascular or mixed neurogenic/vascular impotence.[53] In 144 patients with impotence from various causes, 97% responded positively.[54] Double-blind placebo crossover studies also demonstrate the effectiveness of intracorporal injection of papaverine and phentolamine, and the placebo effect appears to be minimal. In one study of 24 patients, 82.8% had erections after treatments, while no patient who received a saline injection had a positive response.[55] All 18 patients in another study experienced increased penile length and rigidity immediately after injection; although 3 patients who received saline experienced no immediate effect, they reported improved quality of erection over several weeks.[56] In the aforementioned studies, most positive responses resulted in erections sufficient for coitus. Improved quality of erection lasted for several weeks in some patients. If sexual activity closely follows treatment, the psychogenic effect of sexual stimulation may enhance the response to the drugs. A less satisfactory response with increasing age of the patient was observed in one study.[57] Patients with venous leakage should not be given these injections therapeutically, because systemic effects including dizziness, pallor, and sweating have been reported in such individuals after intracavernous papaverine injection.[58]

Various regimens were employed in the aforementioned studies. A mixture of papaverine and phentolamine was injected with a fine-gauge needle into the corpus cavernosum on one side at the base of the penis. Doses ranged from 3 to 30 mg of papaverine plus 0.12 to 1.25 mg of phentolamine administered in a volume of 0.1 to 2 mL (see earlier references). Generally, injection was recommended no more than twice weekly, with the site of injection alternated. Impotence due to various causes appears to respond to papaverine and phentolamine injection, but that due to severe vascular impairment (arterial or venous) is least responsive.[59] Neurogenic impotence responds to the lowest doses of papaverine and phentolamine or to papaverine alone.[53] Reviews of intracavernous injection therapy for impotence, including the selection of patients for whom therapy is appropriate, are available.[60, 61]

Adverse reactions generally are minor and include pain, paresthesia, or bruising or ulcers at the injection site. Prolonged erections are a serious concern and those lasting more than 2 to 4 hours should be treated. If the prolonged erection is painful, indicating ischemia, immediate treatment is indicated. Treatment consists of aspiration of blood or, if that fails, injection of an adrenergic agent. Long-term use of papaverine penile injections may result in Peyronie-like fibrotic plaques at the injection site.[29, 53] One fatality was reported in a paraplegic patient who died from pulmonary thromboembolism presumably caused by papaverine-induced priapism.[62]

Although variations of these methods are widely used and appear to be highly effective, such treatment still must be considered experimental. It is emphasized that experience with this technique is inadequate to assure the safety of long-term therapy. If penile injection of vasoactive agents proves safe and effective, it probably will be used most commonly as an interim measure before the implantation of a penile prosthesis, rather than for long-term treatment.

In a preliminary placebo-controlled, double-blind, crossover study, 8 of 16 impotent men responded positively to oral phentolamine.[63] Further investigation of this oral preparation, which is no longer marked in the United States, is likely.

Penile injection of alprostadil (prostaglandin E_1, PGE_1) has been suggested to improve the quality of erections in patients in whom papaverine has failed or ceased being effective. This agent causes relaxation of smooth muscle and vasodilation. Alprostadil has a shorter duration of action and papaverine, which lessens the likelihood of prolonged erection.[64]

Benign Prostatic Hypertrophy

Benign prostatic hypertrophy accompanied by urinary obstruction is common in aging men. Although it probably occurs in almost 80% of men over 50 years of age, only 10% to 20% experience significant obstruction before 80 years of age. The epithelial and stromal tissues of the prostate enlarge in response to androgenic stimulation. Increased serum and prostate tissue concentration of DHT have been found in these patients compared with unaffected men.[65] Castration or hypopituitarism have been associated with a decrease in prostate size, and surgical resection of the prostate is the current treatment to relieve symptoms.

An effective drug regimen may provide a safer and less expensive alternative to surgery for this condition. Based on known hormonal support of benign prostatic hypertrophy, several approaches to drug treatment have been attempted. Greater symptomatic improvement has occurred in men treated with progestins, Gn-RH analogues, and cyproterone compared with those treated with placebo. Gonadotropin and testosterone secretion are inhibited and, in some patients, prostate size diminishes. Hormonal manipulation appears to be more effective in reducing glandular hyperplasia than primary fibromuscular hyperplasia. However, impotence is a side effect of these methods of medical castration, limiting their usefulness. α-Adrenergic blocking agents such as terazosin or phenoxybenzamine may be effective by producing adrenergic blockade of the smooth muscle at the bladder neck.

Flutamide (Eulexin), a nonsteroidal antiandrogen currently marketed for the treatment of prostate cancer, competes with DHT for androgen receptor sites in the cytosol. When flutamide (750 mg/day) was administered to patients with benign prostatic hypertrophy for 12 weeks and 6 months, prostate volume decreased 18% and 41%, respectively, and uroflow increased 30% and 35%, respectively. No objective improvement was noted with placebo, but symptomatic improvement was comparable in treated and control patients. Side effects in several treated patients included breast pain, gynecomastia, and diarrhea. No patients reported changes in libido or impotence.[66]

Finasteride (MK-906) is an investigational 5α-reductase inhibitor that blocks DHT formation. The plasma testosterone concentration is relatively unaffected, but as with other medical castration therapy, prostate size decreases. However, no adverse effects on libido have been observed.[65]

Micropenis

Micropenis can occur in association with hypospadias, hypogonadotropic or primary hypogonadism, androgen insensitivity, or as an idiopathic condition. Treatment is usually limited to 3 to 6 months to avoid epiphyseal maturation and, ideally, should be undertaken in the neonatal period. Penile growth may occur after the intramuscular administration of testosterone. Alternatively, topical application of testosterone to the penis may be employed, although some authorities feel that that response is better after parenteral administration. It generally is agreed that the action of topical androgen is mediated, at least partly, through systemic absorption of the hormone. It has been suggested that topical application may simplify management and reduce expense. Side effects such as pubic hair development can be minimized by using low concentrations (i.e., 1.25% and 2.5% testosterone).[67] A topical preparation is not available commercially and must be compounded.

Male Contraception

Only two reliable forms of male contraception are available currently in this country: condoms and vasectomy. When used alone, condoms are quite effective; when combined with a vaginal spermicide, the contraceptive efficacy is improved markedly. Because the condom is a mechanical barrier, it also helps to prevent the transmission of sexually transmitted diseases.

Vasectomy is a safe, effective, and economical method to achieve permanent sterility. Other than complications at or soon after surgery (e.g., pain, ecchymosis, infection, granulomas), there are no long-term health risks up to 15 years after vasectomy.[68] Reversibility has been improved markedly by microsurgical vasovasostomy. However, many men who produce an adequate number of sperm postanastomosis remain infertile; the development of antisperm antibodies may be responsible, although their presence is not necessarily associated with infertility.

The pharmacologic approach to male contraception continues to be investigated, but no drugs for this indication are likely to reach the market in the foreseeable future. Pharmacologic agents suppress spermatogenesis through hormonal inhibition of gonadotropin secretion (e.g., Gn-RH or luteinizing hormone releasing hormone [LHRH] analogues, steroids, inhibin), direct inhibition of sperm production without affecting the hormonal milieu (e.g., gossypol),[69] or interference with epididymal maturation of sperm.

Gn-RH analogues act by suppressing the secretion of LH and FSH, which are essential for spermatogenesis. Because LH also is required to stimulate testosterone secretion, libido and potency decreases and secondary sexual characteristics (e.g., beard growth) may be affected adversely. Therefore, to avoid these adverse effects, Gn-RH analogues must be used with testosterone replacement therapy (initially or after azoospermia is achieved). Various steroid agents, including progestins, testosterone, and other androgens, have been used alone or in combination to suppress gonadotropins and hence spermatogenesis. The use of androgens, of course, eliminates the adverse effects on secondary sexual characteristics. Inhibin is a peptide believed to be secreted in the seminiferous tubules by the Sertoli cells, whose function appears to be selective inhibition of FSH secretion by the pituitary. Suppression of FSH secretion probably inhibits spermatogenesis. Inhibin does not influence LH or testosterone secretion.

The main problem with most male contraceptive methods that employ hormonal suppression of spermatogenesis is that the onset and degree of efficacy are inconsistent. Either the dose required for azoospermia is variable or the drug only decreases sperm count, which still may be adequate for fertilization in some men.

Gossypol, a pigment extracted from the cotton plant, directly interferes with spermatogenesis when taken orally. The agent was under investigation in China. Although dramatic reductions in sperm count have been obtained,[70] the high efficacy rates required for marketing a contraceptive agent in the United States may not be achievable. In addition, the prolonged use of gossypol is associated with hypokalemia, which may not be reversible with potassium supplementation[71]; damage to the spermatogenic epithelium may be permanent. Efforts to develop effective male contraceptive methods have been reviewed.[72]

Infertility, General

Almost one half of cases of infertility are at least partially due to reproductive dysfunction in the male partner. Whatever the etiology, male infertility may be manifested by an alteration in sperm density, motility, or morphology or abnormalities of seminal fluid viscosity or volume. The cause may be an anatomic abnormality such as varicocele or cryptorchidism; obstruction of the ductal system due to inflammatory diseases including tuberculosis; gonorrhea; iatrogenic, such as following hernia repair; genetic in cases such as Klinefelter's syndrome; destruction of the germinal epithelium due to such causes as mumps orchitis and irradiation; environmental, such as increased scrotal temperature from hot baths and certain pesticides; immunologic (e.g., sperm antibodies); ejaculatory dysfunction such as retrograde ejaculation; the use of marijuana, which may decrease testosterone levels and cause abnormal spermatogenesis (e.g., motility, morphology, sperm count); acute infection as suggested by leukocytes in the semen; or a side effect of drug therapy (Table 1).[73] Only a small proportion of cases of male infertility is caused by a recognized endocrinologic disorder. Reviews that discuss the causes, diagnosis, and management of male infertility include Sherins and Howards,[74] Griffin,[75] Hirsch and Lipshultz,[76] Bodner,[77] and Spark.[78]

In some cases of male infertility not correctable by drug therapy or surgical intervention, the couple may be suitable candidates for artificial insemination using semen obtained from the husband or a donor. In vitro fertilization may be used for certain patients with male infertility involving low sperm count or motility or abnormal morphology, although the couple should be told that the success rate is likely to be low, especially in the presence of poor morphology. Multiple oocyte retrieval may partially offset low fertilization rates.[79]

TABLE 1.
Effects of Drugs on Male Fertility

Drugs	Reported Effect
Busulfan (Myleran)	Possible sterility, azoospermia, and testicular atrophy
Chlorambucil (Leukeran)	Oligospermia, azoospermia
Cimetidine (Tagamet)	Decreased sperm count
Colchicine	Azoospermia
Cyclophosphamide (Cytoxan, Neosar)	Azoospermia
Diethylstilbestrol (use in pregnancy)	In sons: epididymal cysts, questionable increase in cryptorchidism and infertility
Ethyl alcohol	Decreased serum testosterone, impaired sperm motility
Marijuana	Decreased serum testosterone, decreased sperm count, impaired sperm motility, abnormal morphology
Methadone (Dolophine)	Decreased serum testosterone
Methotrexate (Folex, Mexate)	Oligospermia
Phenytoin (Dilantin)	Decreased follicle-stimulating hormone, oligospermia
Prednisolone	Oligospermia
Spironolactone (Aldactone)	Decreased serum testosterone, increased testosterone clearance
Sulfasalazine (Axulfidine, S.A.S.-500)	Decreased sperm count
Thioridazine (Mellaril)	Slightly decreased serum testosterone

Infertility Due to Varicocele

About 20% to 40% of infertile males are found to have a varicocele, which may contribute to the infertility. Left varicoceles are most common; bilateral involvement occurs less often, and a right varicocele is rare. When left varicocelectomy fails to improve semen quality, further investigation may reveal a right varicocele; if this is corrected, the quality of semen may improve and pregnancy may be achieved.[80] Surgical or venographic correction of venous reflux may be appropriate in patients with oligospermia, which usually is associated with altered motility or morphology. Semen quality may improve in the majority, and pregnancies may be achieved in 30% to 55% of previously childless couples.[81] However, varicoceles also are common in the fertile male population, and some clinicians have questioned the causal relationship between varicoceles and infertility.[82]

Some men in whom sperm density improved postoperatively also showed normalization of hormonal parameters. An exaggerated response to Gn-RH and decreased seminal DHT also were altered toward normal after surgery in some patients. However, patients whose hormonal parameters were normal preoperatively did not experience improvement in sperm density or motility postoperatively, and it was thought that infertility in these men was caused by a factor other than varicocele.[83] This finding was not confirmed by other investigators, who reported improvement in semen quality and fertility in a large series of patients who had normal hormonal parameters preoperatively.[84]

Adjunctive drug therapy with hCG[85, 86] or clomiphene[87, 88] has been suggested for patients with preoperative sperm counts of less than 10 million/mL. However, the efficacy of such regimens remains unproved.

Infertility Due to Hypogonadotropic Hypogonadism

Hypogonadotropic infertility is uncommon. However, spermatogenesis can be initiated and pregnancies achieved in one half of properly selected patients. Definitive diagnostic tests include those that exclude other causes of infertility in both partners; measurement of serum gonadotropins, prolactin, and testosterone; and testicular biopsy.

Hormonal therapy depends on the severity of the defect. When there is only partial gonadotropin deficiency, hCG alone often increases sperm counts and produces normal ejaculates. In patients with severe deficiency, androgen therapy stimulates virilization during adolescence. Because maximum stimulation of spermatogenesis may require 1 year of gonadotropin replacement, androgen therapy may be discontinued and the administration of gonadotropin begun when the patient reaches his early twenties. Alternatively, gonadotropin therapy may be postponed until the patient desires fertility.

In complete hypogonadotropic hypogonadism, hCG stimulates testicular development only partially despite complete virilization. After normal serum testosterone levels are achieved and there is no further increase in testicular growth or improvement in sperm production, menotropins is added to the regimen (see the evaluations). After successful treatment, most patients with complete hypogonadotropic hypogonadism achieve adequate testicular size and produce ejaculates containing 2 to 5 million or more sperm per milliliter. Pregnancies have occurred at this low sperm level when the female partner has normal fertility. When maximal stimulation of germinal tissue and sperm output has been achieved, menotropins is withdrawn. Spermatogenesis is maintained by the continued administration of hCG,[89] although a study in normal males suggests that FSH activity (present in menotropins but not in hCG) is necessary to support the production of normal numbers of sperm.[90] In men with only partial gonadotropin deficiency, hCG alone stimulated the completion of spermatogenesis, and the degree of response correlated with the size of the testis before treatment (i.e., the least impaired subjects demonstrated the best response). Pregnancies were achieved with average sperm counts of only 8.7 million/mL.[91]

Studies have shown that infertile men with hypogonadotropic hypogonadism can be treated successfully by the pulsatile administration of Gn-RH,[92, 93] but the optimal dose and frequency of administration have not been determined. Gn-RH therapy, which requires the presence of an intact pituitary offers the appealing possibility of correcting the gonadotropin abnormality with a more physiologic pattern of endogenous gonadotropin secretion than is possible with exogenous administration of gonadotropins. The pulsatile administration of Gn-RH simulates the physiologic condition where Gn-RH stimulates gonadotropin secretion. This is in marked contrast to the effect of long-acting Gn-RH analogues, which, after initial stimulation, result in down-regulation of receptors and decreased gonadotropin secretion. Pulsatile Gn-RH, which can be administered using a portable infusion pump, may be preferable to treatment with an hCG-menotropins regimen, which requires several injections weekly. The dose, frequency of the pulse, and total amount of hormone administered can affect the differential pattern of gonadotropin secretion. For example, longer pulse intervals appear to enhance FSH secretion.[94] Other evidence suggests that pulses every 2 hours may be optimal for LH secretion.[95] Gn-RH pulse parameters also may affect the biologic:immunologic activity ratio of the LH secreted.[96] Relatively high serum production (96 million/mL) has been reported when Gn-RH was used to treat infertility in hypogonadotropic hypogonadism.[97]

The administration of Gn-RH by the intranasal route also is being investigated. Doses 50 to 100 times greater than those used for intravenous administration are given every 2 hours except during sleep.[98]

Infertility Due to Hyperprolactinemia

Since both men and women require gonadotropic support for gametogenesis, it seems reasonable to expect that the male as well as the female reproductive system may be subject to various inhibitions associated with elevated prolactin levels. Galactorrhea sometimes occurs in males with prolactin-secreting tumors, and impotence is often, but not invariably, present. Hyperprolactinemia may account for refractoriness in some men whose hormonal profiles indicate that they are candidates for clomiphene or hCG therapy. In some men, LH concentration and pulse frequency, sperm counts, and testosterone levels are increased following the use of bromocriptine to normalize serum prolactin levels.[99] The identification and treatment of selected patients with bromocriptine may improve pregnancy rates in patients who otherwise would be treatment "failures," but the efficacy of this treatment has not been confirmed.

Idiopathic Male Infertility

Probably 40% to 60% of all infertile males have no identifiable anatomic or endocrine defect. Therapy in these cases is empiric and nonspecific. Clomiphene is commonly employed to treat subfertile males (see the evaluation). However, the lack of controlled studies, standardized patient selection, and treatment regimens makes the interpretation of clinical results difficult; consequently, this therapy is not endorsed by all experts, and the use and effectiveness of clomiphene therapy in male infertility remain controversial. Lack of effectiveness was reported in a placebo-controlled study in which clomiphene was administered to men with oligospermia and normal hormonal levels. After clomiphene therapy, although gonadotropin and testosterone levels and gonadotropin secretory response to Gn-RH were increased, no improvement in semen parameters, results of sperm penetration assay, or pregnancy rate was observed.[100]

As in women, clomiphene stimulates endogenous gonadotropin secretion. Criteria for patient selection include serum gonadotropin and testosterone levels usually within the normal range. If a testicular biopsy is performed, it may indicate the presence of all germinal elements, although decreased in number (hypospermatogenesis). Clomiphene usually increases serum testosterone levels and occasionally may increase the number and motility of sperm. Clomiphene therapy should be withdrawn after 6 months if there has been no improvement in semen quality, if a marked rise in the FSH or testosterone level occurs, or if there is worsening of the semen quality after earlier improvement.

Successful treatment of some men with idiopathic infertility was reported in an uncontrolled study using tamoxifen (Nolvadex), another antiestrogenic agent[101]; however, the initial increase in sperm count may be followed by a decline. In a later report, tamoxifen was found to be no more effective than placebo for this indication.[102] Patients with primary testicular failure (increased serum FSH, hyalinization, or other evidence of permanent epithelial damage) or ductal obstruction are not suitable candidates for gonadotropin or gonadotropin-stimulating therapy.[103]

Gonadotropins (hCG or a combination of hCG and menotropins) also have been used investigationally to treat idiopathic male infertility, particularly that unresponsive to clomiphene. Although success has been reported in some men,[86, 104] results generally have been disappointing. The necessity for repeated intramuscular injections is inconvenient, and treatment, particularly when menotropins is employed, is expensive. The effectiveness of gonadotropin therapy in males with a normal sperm count is doubtful.

Testosterone rebound has been employed sporadically since its introduction 30 years ago. A depot preparation (testosterone enanthate or cypionate 200 mg) is injected intramuscularly once weekly for 12 to 20 weeks. The negative feedback effect of testosterone suppresses pituitary gonadotropin output and azoospermia ensues. Following the cessation of therapy, there have been some reports of a rebound phenomenon in which the germinal epithelium recovers function and sperm production is increased to a level compatible with fertility. The action has been ascribed to the release of gonadotropin that was stored in the pituitary during the period of testosterone suppression. Success rates are variable but do not exceed 20%, and there are several disadvantages. First, the treatment period is long and rebound sperm production is delayed for 3 to 4 months after the cessation of therapy. Second, in most men, the improvement in sperm production lasts only 2 to 3 months. Third, treatment may be followed by permanent depression of the sperm count.[105] Because of these problems and the uncertainty of success, the testosterone suppression method is best reserved for patients with severe idiopathic oligospermia who do not respond to other therapy and who understand the possible consequences of treatment.

In the past, thyroid and adrenal supplements were used empirically; however, more sensitive diagnostic endocrine tests are available today, and such treatment cannot be recommended unless thyroid or adrenal hormone deficiency has been documented. In uncontrolled studies, improved sperm motility with an increase in the number of pregnancies has been reported following the administration of low doses of androgen to infertile males with a defect of sperm motility but normal sperm counts, morphology, and serum testosterone levels.[106] Prolonged administration may result in decreased sperm counts, and this use of testosterone now is not generally recommended.

Infertile men with poor sperm motility and low seminal zinc concentration responded more favorably to the administration of zinc and fluoxymesterone (Halotestin) than to either agent alone. However, pregnancy rates were not reported.[107] The prostaglandin inhibitory effect of some anti-inflammatory drugs is postulated to cause improved sperm quality in oligospermic infertile men,[108] but this has not been confirmed. In the presence of infection, appropriate antibiotic therapy may be effective.[109]

Immunologic Infertility

Antibodies to sperm in the semen or in the female reproductive tract may cause infertility. Antibodies present on sperm or in the cervical mucus may prevent the penetration or progress of sperm in the cervical mucus that results in an abnormal postcoital test. Less frequently, sperm antibodies can interfere directly with fertilization. Antibodies directed at the head or main tailpiece may affect fertility. Antibody testing is suggested for those couples in whom both an abnormal postcoital test and normal semen analysis are found, or when there is spontaneous microscopic agglutination of sperm in the semen. Infertility due to sperm antibodies may affect one third of patients who have had vasovasostomy following vasectomy.[110, 111]

Attempts to treat infertility caused by sperm antibodies are often unsuccessful, but several options are available. When the female partner is affected, the use of a condom reduces exposure to sperm antigens and may decrease antibody levels. Unprotected coitus at the time of ovulation then may be successful. When the male partner develops autoimmunity to sperm, the semen can be washed to remove antibodies and then used for insemination. However, this technique has not been particularly helpful. Alternatively, artificial insemination of donor semen may be attempted.

Immunosuppressive therapy with large doses of corticosteroids (prednisolone 60 mg/day for 7 or 14 days) also has been suggested.[112] Pregnancies were achieved within 4 months in 45% of treated couples compared to 12% of untreated couples. Regimens using larger amounts of corticosteroids have been reported.[113] The couple must weigh the possibility of adverse effects from this experimental treatment (e.g., effects on carbohydrate and lipid metabolism and central nervous system function; electrolyte changes; negative nitrogen balance; osteoporosis; osteonecrosis; myopathy) against the importance of a possible pregnancy.[114]

Androgenic Agents

This section addresses the aforementioned topics as applied to most therapeutic uses of androgens.

Adverse Reactions and Precautions

When androgens are administered to prepubertal boys, virilism may occur. Signs of virilism in prepubertal children are pubic hair development, phallic enlargement, and increased frequency of erections. There is a risk of priapism; any increase in erectile frequency is an indication for reducing the dose. In aging men, androgens may stimulate prostatic hyperplasia, causing urinary obstruction. Paradoxically, androgens may cause gynecomastia, particularly in children (e.g., when used for constitutional delay of growth), or in men after the administration of large doses or in the presence of liver disease. This probably is due to the aromatization of testosterone to estrogen and does not occur with the use of steroids that are reduced in the 5α position.

Androgens and anabolic steroids (weak androgens designed to provide anabolic activity with little androgenic effect) should not be used to stimulate growth in children who are small but otherwise normal and healthy, except in selected cases of constitutional delayed growth. When they are used, the rate of skeletal maturation may exceed the rate of linear growth, thereby inducing premature closure of the epiphyses and reducing the attainable adult height. The extent to which this complication occurs depends on the child's bone age, the drug used, the dosage, and the duration of therapy. The decision to administer anabolic steroids to children for a specific growth problem should be made only after careful evaluation by an experienced pediatric endocrinologist.

Androgenic and anabolic steroids with an alkyl group substituted in the alpha position on carbon 17 (i.e., methyltestosterone [Metandren, Oreton Methyl, Testred], fluoxymesterone [Halotestin], ethylestrenol [Maxibolin], methandrostenolone (no longer marketed in the United States), oxandrolone [Anavar], oxymetholone [Anadrol-50], stanozolol [Winstrol]), as well as the impeded androgen, danazol (Danocrine), have produced signs of liver dysfunction. Increased sulfobromophthalein retention and serum glutamic oxaloacetic transaminase levels appear to be dose-related and are relatively unimportant. Increased serum bilirubin and alkaline phosphatase values indicating excretory dysfunction are rare but important idiosyncratic reactions. Clinical jaundice is unusual and reversible when the drug is discontinued. The histologic findings consist of intrahepatic cholestasis with little or no cellular damage. Therefore, these drugs should be used with caution in all patients and particularly in those with preexisting liver disease. Long-term administration of 17 α-alkylated androgens and anabolic steroids should be avoided.

Rarely, hepatocellular and endothelial malignancies, hepatic adenomas, and intrahepatic hemorrhage associated with peliosis hepatis, have developed, particularly in anemic patients treated for long periods with large doses of 17 α-alkylated steroids. Hepatocellular adenomas or carcinomas may regress when androgens are discontinued. Patients with Fanconi's syndrome experience more severe liver toxicity from androgen therapy than do other patients with anemia; it is not known whether this is due to prolonged androgen therapy or increased susceptibility to liver dysfunction in these patients.[115] Patients receiving prolonged androgen therapy should be monitored for functional and structural liver abnormalities.

Abnormal liver function tests are thought to occur less frequently with intramuscular preparations of testosterone and its derivatives and nandrolone phenpropionate and decanoate, which lack the 17 α-alkylated group. Large doses of androgens and anabolic steroids, such as those taken by some athletes for body-building purposes, can cause potentially atherogenic changes in blood lipids.[116]

Salt and fluid retention are usually not serious but can be undesirable in elderly patients, those with congestive heart failure, or those with a tendency to develop edema from other causes (e.g., cirrhosis, hypoproteinemia). Care should be taken when 17 α-alkylated preparations are used in patients on hemodialysis, because these drugs may increase blood fibrinolytic activity. Androgens are contraindicated in men with carcinoma of the prostate or breast.

Drug Interactions

When an androgen is administered to patients taking an oral anticoagulant, the activity of the latter is enhanced and severe bleeding episodes may occur. The anticoagulant dose may have to be reduced to 25% of that appropriate for use without androgen. The mechanism of the increased hypoprothrombinemic response is undetermined. The effect occurs rapidly, within several days to a week, and usually reverses in a similar pattern when androgen is discontinued. This interaction is known to occur with 17 α-alkylated androgens and also may occur with testosterone.[117] Therefore, when any androgenic steroid is added to or withdrawn from a regimen that also includes an anticoagulant, more frequent prothrombin determinations and adjustments in dose of the anticoagulant should be made.

Methandrostenolone may decrease the metabolism of oxyphenbutazone, resulting in a longer, more intense, and unpredictable response to the latter. Therefore, it is advisable to avoid the concomitant use of these drugs. Methandrostenolone also has been reported to increase both the therapeutic and toxic effects of corticosteroids. The requirement for antidiabetic agents may be decreased when anabolic steroids are added to the regimen, because the latter may reduce blood sugar levels directly in diabetics.

Glucocorticoids depress the level of endogenous serum testosterone. The probable mechanism is suppression of hypothalamic Gn-RH secretion. When conditions such as impotence or osteopenia occur in men treated for prolonged periods with glucocorticoids, they may be related to decreased serum testosterone rather than to the illness per se.[118]

Effects on Laboratory Tests

Androgens reduce the level of circulating thyroxine-binding globulin, thereby decreasing thyroid hormone levels and increasing triiodothyronine resin uptake. However, the free triiodothyronine and thyroxine are unaffected and there is no evidence of thyroid dysfunction. Androgens enhance blood fibrinolytic activity, increase hematocrit and serum haptoglobin levels, and have variable effects on serum lipids. The administration of testosterone, but not the 17 α-alkylated derivatives, elevates urinary 17-ketosteroids.

Preparations

Unaltered testosterone is not suitable for oral or parenteral administration because absorption and hepatic degradation are rapid. Esterification of testosterone has produced molecules that are less polar and are soluble in oil vehicles and fatty tissue. Generally, the longer the carbon chain of the ester substituent, the more slowly the hormone is released into the circulation. The esters are hydrolyzed to testosterone, which can be assayed in the blood when monitoring therapy. Testosterone esters are administered as the propionate, cypionate (Andro-Cyp, Depo-Testosterone), and enanthate (Andryl, Delatestryl). Testosterone propionate is injected two to four times weekly, while the longer-acting cypionate and enanthate are administered every 2 to 4 weeks. The latter two preparations are drugs of choice for hypogonadism, which requires long-term therapy.

Methyltestosterone (Metandren, Oreton Methyl, Testred) and fluoxymesterone (Halotestin) are alkyalted in the 17 α position, which retards hepatic degradation and renders these preparations effective after oral administration. They must be given daily and their androgenic potency, milligram-for-milligram, is less than that of the parenteral forms of testosterone. Also, 17 α-alkylated androgens may be more hepatotoxic (see the discussion on adverse reactions and precautions).

Newer preparations that provide greater ease of administration and effectiveness are being developed. Siloxane capsules containing testosterone are implanted subcutaneously and provide relatively constant blood levels over a long period. An investigational transdermal system consisting of testosterone-impregnated adhesive film also is being tested, and results have been promising (see the section on hyogonadism earlier). The undecanoate ester of testosterone (marketed in other countries) and a preparation of microparticulate testosterone that are effective orally also are being investigated.

Drug Evaluations

Androgens

Fluoxymesterone.—Fluoxymesterone is a short-acting preparation (with a half-life of about 10 hours) that is used orally. It is less effective for replacement therapy than the long-acting esters of testosterone. Full sexual maturation in patients with prepubertal hypogonadism cannot be achieved easily with fluoxymesterone, but it is used sometimes for replacement therapy when hypogonadism begins in adult life or after secondary sexual characteristics have developed following therapy with a parenteral preparation. However, because of its potential hepatotoxicity, this androgen should not be used for long periods.

See the general discussion on androgens for information on other indications and adverse reactions. For androgen deficiency, fluoxymesterone is given orally at a dose of 10 to 20 mg daily. It is available in generic form or as the brand Halotestin (Upjohn), in tablets of 2, 5, and 10 mg.

Methyltestosterone.—Methyltestosterone is a short-acting preparation (with a half-life of about 2.5 hours) that is used orally and buccally. Although absorption is more variable, the bioavailability is greater with buccal administration, probably because the hepatic circulation is bypassed. However, the oral route is used more commonly for convenience.

Methyltestosterone is much less effective for replacement therapy than are the long-acting esters of testosterone. Although methyltestosterone does not produce full sexual maturation in patients with prepubertal hypogonadism, it is used sometimes for replacement therapy when hypogonadism begins in adult life or after secondary sexual characteristics have developed following therapy with testosterone. However, because of its potential hepatotoxicity, this androgen should not be used for long periods.

For androgen deficiency, methyltestosterone is given orally at a dose of 10 to 50 mg daily. It is available in generic form or as the brands Metandren (CIBA) and Oreton Methyl (Schering) in tablets of 10 and 25 mg or the brand Testred (ICN) in capsules of 10 mg. Methyltestosterone is administered buccally in adults at one half of the oral dosage (the rate of absorption is variable). It is available in generic form or as the Metandren (CIBA) in tablets (buccal) of 5 and 10 mg or the brand Oreton Methyl (Schering) in tablets (buccal) of 10 mg.

Testosterone Cypionate and Testosterone Enanthate.—Testosterone cypionate and enanthate are long-acting, potent esters of testosterone given intramuscularly to develop or maintain secondary sexual characteristics and other physiologic functions in androgen-deficient males. These agents are preferred to induce full sexual development in eunuchoidal males when testicular disease has interfered with normal pubertal development and to treat postpubertal Leydig cell failure. Peak blood levels are achieved within 1 day after administration and decline to baseline levels after 7 to 9 days, depending on the dose. Thus, intramuscular administration of these preparations results in uneven serum levels of testosterone, and it is recommended that the dosing interval not exceed 2 to 3 weeks to avoid long periods without androgen support.[67] These preparations also may be given to initiate puberty in selected boys with constitutional delay of growth.

Intramuscular dosing is as follows. For the induction of puberty in boys, 50 mg/m^2/month closely simulates the first year of puberty; 100 mg/m^2 /month simulates normal midpuberty sexual development and growth spurt. The following regimen is suggested: 50 mg is given every 4 weeks to accomplish growth, followed the second or third year by 100 mg every 4 weeks. The dosage is increased gradually thereafter to the following maintenance schedule for adults. For androgen deficiency, 100 mg/m^2, 150 to 200 mg every 2 weeks, or 300 mg every 3 weeks is given.

Testosterone cypionate is available in generic form as a solution (in oil) of 100 and 200 mg/mL in 10-mL containers. It is also available as the brand Andro-Cyp (Keene) as a solution (in cottonseed oil) of 100 and 200 mg/mL in 1- and 10-mL containers or as the brand Depo-Testosterone (Upjohn) as a solution (in cottonseed oil) of 100 and 200 mg/mL in 1- and 10/mL containers.

Testosterone enanthate is available in generic form as a solution (in oil) of 100 and 200 mg/mL in 5- and 10-mL containers. It is also available as the brand Andryl (Keene) as a solution (in sesame oil) of 200 mg/mL in 10-mL containers or as the brand Delatestryl (Squibb-Mark) as a solution (in sesame oil) of 200 mg/mL in 1- and 5-mL containers.

Testosterone Propionate.—Testosterone propionate can be used to induce or maintain secondary sexual characteristics and other physiologic functions in androgen-deficient males. This relatively short-acting preparation produces a steady response when used parenterally, but this route is not practical for long-term therapy. In older patients, the prostate gland may be sensitive to androgen and bladder neck obstruction may develop; this complication is corrected more easily if a short-acting preparation is used initially.

Intramuscular dosing for androgen deficiency is 50 mg three times weekly. Testosterone propionate is available in generic form as a solution (in oil) of 25 mg/mL in 10-mL containers and 50 and 100 mg/mL in 10- and 30-mL containers.

Anterior Pituitary and Hypothalamic Agents

Bromocriptine Mesylate.—The usefulness of this semisynthetic ergot alkaloid depends primarily on its dopaminergic activity. Bromocriptine inhibits the secretion of prolactin by the anterior pituitary gland. Impotence, hypogonadism, or infertility in males associated with elevated prolactin levels sometimes responds to bromocriptine. The drug is not effective in psychogenic impotence or that caused by conditions other than hyperprolactinemia. Symptoms frequently recur upon cessation of therapy.

The doses employed for reproductive dysfunction generally do not cause severe side effects. Nausea is most common, but vomiting, constipation, dizziness, and orthostatic hypotension also occur. These effects can be minimized by taking the medication with food and at bedtime and by initiating therapy with small doses and gradually increasing the amount to effective levels.

Bromocriptine should be taken with food. The oral dose in appropriately selected males with elevated plasma prolactin is 2.5 mg twice daily. It is available as the brand Parlodel (Sandoz) in capsules of 5 mg and tablets of 2.5 mg.

Clomiphene Citrate.—This nonsteroidal agent is a mixture of two isomers in approximately a 1:1 ratio and is related chemically to chlorotrianisene. It sometimes is used to stimulate sperm production in selected males with idiopathic infertility.

For oligospermia in selected males, an oral dose of 25 mg daily is commonly used. Alternatively, 100 mg is given every other day or three times a week.[119] Medication is continued for 6 to 12 months or until pregnancy is achieved. Clomiphene citrate is available as the brands Clomid (Merrell Dow) and Serophene (Serono) in tablets of 50 mg.

Human Chorionic Gonadotropin.—hCG is a placental hormone extracted from the urine of pregnant women. Its biological activity is the same as that of LH and it is used as a substitute for human LH, which accounts for the thyrotoxic state that occurs in patients with hCG-secreting neoplasms. This preparation sometimes is used diagnostically in males with delayed puberty or when there is doubt about the steroidogenic ability of the testes to respond to gonadotropin stimulation. hCG also is used to treat cryptorchidism in selected males and to treat infertility in males with hypogonadotropic hypogonadism. hCG stimulates or maintains spermatogenesis depending on the hormonal status of the patient and the regimen used.

The intramuscular dose is as follows. In cryptorchidism, for rapid response and minimal sexual development, 5,000 units is given every 3 to 4 days for four injections; to achieve a greater degree of sexual development, 500 units is given three times weekly for 3 weeks or, for boys 10 years or older, 1,000 units is given twice weekly for 3 weeks. In males, for diagnosis of responsiveness to gonadotropin stimulation, 5,000 units is given once. Blood levels of testosterone are measured before treatment and 3 to 4 days later. An approximate doubling of testosterone levels is normal.[120]

For hypogonadotropic infertility in men, 2,000 units is given two or three times a week. When normal serum testosterone levels are reached and there is no further testicular growth or improvement in sperm production, menotropins may be added to the regimen. When maximal spermatogenesis is established, sperm production usually continues as long as hCG (2,000 units three times a week) is given. hCG is available in generic form or as the brand A.P.L. (Ayerst) in a powder of 5,000, 10,000, and 20,000 USP units with 10 mL of diluent. It is also available as Follutein (Squibb) and Pregnyl (Organon) in a powder (lyophilized) of 10,000 USP units with 10 mL of diluent or as the brand Profasi HP (Serono) in a powder (sterile, lyophilized) of 5,000 and 10,000 USP units with 10 mL of diluent.

Menotropins.—Menotropins is a preparation of human menopausal gonadotropin extracted from the urine of postmenopausal women. FSH and LH activity are present in a 1:1 ratio. The goal of therapy in males is to replace gonadotropins and stimulate spermatogenesis. Menotropins is sometimes used with hCG to treat hypogonadotropic male infertility, and it has been used investigationally in idiopathic male infertility. Such treatment is prolonged and expensive.

The intramuscular dose is as follows. For hypogonadotropic or idiopathic male infertility (to be given with hCG; see the evaluation on hCG), 75 IU is given three times a week. (One half of patients respond to 25 IU three times per week. Therefore, lower dosages may be tried.) Effectiveness of therapy is determined after 6 to 9 months at a specific dosage level. When maximal stimulation of the germinal tissue and sperm output has been achieved, menotropins can be discontinued; sperm production continues as long as hCG (2,000 units three times a week) is given. Menotropins is available as the brand Pergonal (Serono) in a solution containing 75 or 150 IU each of FSH activity and LH activity (with 10 mg of lyophilized lactose) in 2-mL containers.

References

1. Burger HG, McLachlan RI, Bangah M, et al: Serum inhibin concentrations rise throughout normal male and female puberty. *J Clin Endocrinol Metab* 1988; 67:689–694.
2. De Jong FH: Inhibin. *Physiol Rev* 1988; 68:555–607.
3. Neaves WB, Johnson L, Porter JC, et al: Leydig cell numbers, daily sperm production, and serum gonadotropin levels in aging men. *J Clin Endocrinol Metab* 1984; 59:756–763.
4. Nankin HR, Calkins JH: Decreased bioavailable testosterone in aging normal and impotent men. *J Clin Endocrinol Metab* 1986; 63:1418–1420.
5. Davidson JM, Chen JJ, Crapo L, et al: Hormonal changes and sexual function in aging men. *J Clin Endocrinol Metab* 1983; 57:71–77.
6. Magee MC: Physiology of sexual behavior: Embryologic organization and adult activation. *Urology* 1983; 22:467–478.
7. Gorski RA, Lippe BM, Green R: Androgens and sexual behavior. *Ann Intern Med* 96:488–501.
8. Gladue RA, Green R, Hellman RE: Neuroendocrine response to estrogen and sexual orientation. *Science* 1984; 225:1496–1499.
9. Gooren L: Neuroendocrine response of luteinizing hormone to estrogen administration in heterosexual, homosexual, and transsexual subjects. *J Clin Endocrinol Metab* 1986; 63:583–588.
10. Wagner IOF, Brabant G, Warsch F, et al: Pulsatile gonadotropin-releasing hormone treatment in idiopathic delayed puberty. *J Clin Endocrinol Metab* 1986; 62:95–102.
11. Rosenfeld RG, Northcraft GB, Hintz RL: Prospective, randomized study of testosterone treatment of constitutional delay of growth and development in male adolescence. *Pediatrics* 1982; 69:681–687.
12. Kelley VC, Ruvalcaba RHA: Use of anabolic agents in treatment of short children. *J Clin Endocrinol Metab* 1982; 11:25–39.
13. Kulin HE: Delayed puberty in the male, in Krieger DT, Bardin CW (eds): *Current Therapy in Endocrinology 1983–1984.* Toronto, Canada, BC Decker Inc, 1983, pp 351–354.
14. Elder JS: Cryptorchidism: Isolated and associated with other genitourinary defects. *Pediatr Adolesc Endocrinol* 1987; 34:1033–1053.
15. Depue RH, Pike MC, Henderson BE: Cryptorchidism and testicular cancer (letter). *J Natl Cancer Inst* 1986; 77:830–833.
16. Strader CH, Weiss NS, Daling JR, et al: Cryptorchism, orchiopexy, and the risk of testicular cancer. *Am J Epidemiol* 1988; 127:1013–1018.
17. Chilvers C, Dudley NE, Gough MH, et al: Undescended testis: Effect of treatment on subsequent risk of subfertility and malignancy. *J Pediatr Surg* 1986; 21:691–696.
18. Pike MC, Chilvers C, Peckham MJ: Effect of age at orchidopexy on risk of testicular cancer. *Lancet* 1986; 1:1246–1248.
19. Pottern LM, Brown LM, Hoover RN, et al: Testicular cancer risk among young men: Role of cryptorchidism and inguinal hernia. *J Natl Cancer Inst* 1985; 74:377–381.
20. Rajfer J, Handelsman DJ, Swerdloff RS, et al: Hormonal therapy of cryptorchidism: Randomized, double-blind study comparing human chorionic gonadotropin and gonadotropin-releasing hormone. *J Engl J Med* 1986; 314:466–470.

21. de Muinck Keizer-Schrama SMPF, Hazebroek FWJ, Matroos AW, et al: Double-blind, placebo-controlled study of luteinizing hormone-releasing hormone nasal spray in treatment of undescended testes. *Lancet* 1986; 1:876–880.
22. Chilvers C, Jackson MB, Pike MC: Luteinizing-hormone-releasing hormone and cryptorchidism (letter). *Lancet* 1986; 1:101.
23. Spratt DI, Carr DB, Merriam GR, et al: Spectrum of abnormal patterns of gonadotropin-releasing hormone secretion in men with idiopathic hypogonadotropic hypogonadism: Clinical and laboratory correlations. *J Clin Endocrinol Metab* 1987; 64:283–291.
24. Korenman SG, Viosca S, Garza D, et al: Androgen therapy of hypogonadal men with transcrotal testosterone systems. *Am J Med* 1987; 83:471–478.
25. Findlay JC, Place V, Snyder PJ: Treatment of primary hypogonadism in men by the transdermal administration of testosterone. *J Clin Endocrinol Metab* 1989; 68:369–373.
26. Ahmed SR, Boucher AE, Manni A, et al: Transdermal testosterone therapy in the treatment of male hypogonadism. *J Clin Endocrinol Metab* 1988; 66:546–551.
27. Cunningham GR, Cordero E, Thornby JI: Testosterone replacement with transdermal therapeutic systems: Phsyiological serum testosterone and elevated dihydrotestosterone levels. *JAMA* 1989; 261:2525–2530.
28. Lue TF, Tanagho EA: Physiology of erection and pharmacological management of impotence. *J Urol* 1987; 173:829–836.
29. Malloy TR, Malkowicz B: Pharmacologic treatment of impotence. *Urol Clin North Am* 1987; 14:297–305.
30. Buffum J: Pharmacosexology update: Prescription drugs and sexual function. *J Psychoactive Drugs* 1986; 18:97–106.
31. Drugs that cause sexual dysfunction. *Med Lett Drugs Ther* 1987; 29:65–70.
32. McWaine DE, Procci WR: Drug-induced sexual dysfunction. *Med Toxicol Adverse Drug Exp* 1988; 3:289–306.
33. Kaiser FE, Korenman SG: Impotence in diabetic men. *Am J Med* 1988; 85(suppl 5A):147–152.
34. Johnson LE, Morley JE: Impotence in the elderly. *Am Fam Physician* 1988; 38:225–240.
35. Bradley WE: New techniques in evaluation of impotence. *Urology* 1987; 29:383–386.
36. Barry JM, Blank B, Boileau M: Nocturnal penile tumescence monitoring with stamps. *Urology* 1980; 15:171–172.
37. Abber JC, Lue TF, Orvis BR, et al: Diagnostic tests for impotence: Comparison of papaverine injection with the penile-brachial index and nocturnal penile tumescence monitoring. *J Urol* 1986; 135:923–925.
38. Buvat J, Buvat-Herbaut M, Dehaene JL, et al: Is intracavernous injection of papaverine a reliable screening test for vascular impotence? *J Urol* 1986; 135:476–482.
39. Mueller SC, Lue TF: Evaluation of vasculogenic impotence. *Urol Clin North Am* 1988; 15:65–76.
40. Padma-Nathan H: Neurologic evaluation of erectile dysfunction. *Urol Clin North Am* 1988; 15:77–80.
41. McClure RD: Endocrine evaluation and therapy of erectile dysfunction. *Urol Clin North Am* 1988; 15:53–64.
42. Krauss DJ: Management of impotence, II: Selected surgical procedures: Penile prostheses. *Clin Ther* 1987; 9:149–156.

43. Orvis BR, Lue TF: New therapy for impotence. *Urol Clin North Am* 1987; 14:569–581.
44. Murray FT, Wyss HU, Thomas RG, et al: Gonadal dysfunction in diabetic men with organic impotence. *J Clin Endocrinol Metab* 1987; 65:127–135.
45. Meares EM: Testosterone for impotence (letter). *JAMA* 1987; 257:3284.
46. Morales A, Surridge DHC, Marshall PG, et al: Nonhormonal pharmacological treatment of organic impotence. *J Urol* 1982; 128:45–47.
47. Morales A, Condra M, Owen JA, et al: Is yohimbine effective in treatment of organic impotence? Results of controlled trial. *J Urol* 1987; 137:1168–1172.
48. Reid K, Morales A, Harris C, et al: Double-blind trial of yohimbine in treatment of psychogenic impotence. *Lancet* 1987; 2:421–423.
49. Buffam J: Pharmacosexology update: Yohimbine and sexual function. *J Psychoactive Drugs* 1985; 17:131–132.
50. Yohimbine: Time for resurrection? *Lancet* 1986; 2:1194–1195.
51. Brindley GS: Cavernosal alpha-blockade: New technique for investigating and treating erectile impotence. *Br J Psychiatry* 1983; 143:332–337.
52. Janosko EO: Intracavernous self-injection of papaverine and Regitine for the treatment of organic impotence. *N C Med J* 1986; 47:305–307.
53. Sidi AA, Cameron JS, Duffy LM, et al: Intracavernous drug-induced erections in the management of male erectile dysfunction: Experience with 100 patients. *J Urol* 1986; 135:704–706.
54. Robinette MA, Moffat MJ: Intracorporal injection of papaverine and phentolamine in the management of impotence. *Br J Urol* 1986; 58:692–695.
55. Gasser TC, Roach RM, Larsen EH, et al: Intracavernous self-injection with phentolamine and papaverine for the treatment of impotence. *J Urol* 1987; 137:678–680.
56. Kiely EA, Ignotus P, Williams G: Penile function following intracavernosal injection of vasoactive agents or saline. *Br J Urol* 1987; 59:473–476.
57. Strachan JR, Pryor JP: Diagnostic intracorporeal papaverine and erectile dysfunction. *Br J Urol* 1987; 59:264–266.
58. Wespes E, Schulman CC: Systemic complication of intracavernous papaverine injection in patients with venous leakage. *Urology* 1988; 31:114–115.
59. Nellans RE, Ellis LR, Kramer-Levien D: Pharmacological erection: Diagnosis and treatment applications in 69 patients. *J Urol* 1987; 138:52–54.
60. Kursh ED, Bodner DR, Resnick MI, et al: Injection therapy for impotence. *Urol Clin North Am* 1988; 15:625–629.
61. Sidi AA: Vasoactive intracavernous pharmacotherapy. *Urol Clin North Am* 1988; 15:95–101.
62. Hashmat AI, Abraham J: Papaverine induced priapism: Lethal complication (abstract). *Urology* 1987; 37:201A.
63. Gwinup G: Oral phentolamine in non-specific erectile insufficiency. *Ann Intern Med* 1988; 109:162–163.
64. Reiss H: Use of prostaglandin E_1 for papaverine-failed erections. *Urology* 1989; 33:15–16.
65. Geller J: Overview of benign prostatic hypertrophy. *Urology* 1989; 34(suppl):57–63.
66. Stone NN: Flutamide in treatment of benign prostatic hypertrophy. *Urology* 1988; 34(suppl):64–68.
67. Sokol RZ, Swerdloff RS: Hypogonadism: Androgen therapy, in Krieger DT, Bardin GW (eds): *Current Therapy in Endocrinology 1983–1984.* Toronto, Canada, BG Decker Inc, 1983, pp 345–351.

68. Rosenberg L, Schwingl PJ, Kaufman DW, et al: Risk of myocardial infarction 10 or more years after vasectomy in men under 55 years of age. *Am J Epidemiol* 1986; 123:1049–1056.
69. Waites GMH: Male fertility regulation: Recent advances. *Bull WHO* 1986; 64:151–158.
70. Liu G-z, Lyle KC, Cao J: Clinical trial of gossypol as a male contraceptive drug, Part I: Efficacy study. *Fertil Steril* 1987; 48:459–461.
71. Liu G-z, Lyle KC: Clinical trial of gossypol as male contraceptive drug, Part II: Hypokalemia study. *Fertil Steril* 1987; 48:462–465.
72. Wu FGW: Male contraception: Current status and future prospects. *Clin Endocrinol (Oxf)* 1988; 29:443–465.
73. Drife JO: Effects of drugs on sperm. *Drugs* 1987; 33:610–622.
74. Sherins RJ, Howards SS: Male infertility, in Walsh PG, Gilles RF, Perlmutter AD, et al (eds): *Campbell's Urology,* vol 1, ed 5. Philadelphia, WB Saunders, 1986, pp 640–697.
75. Griffin JE: Diagnosis and management of male infertility. *Adv Intern Med* 1987; 32:259–282.
76. Hirsch IH, Lipshultz LI: Medical treatment of male infertility. *Urol Clin North Am* 1987; 14:307–322.
77. Bodner DR: Critical review of pharmacologic therapies. *Semin Reprod Endocrinol* 1988; 6:377–384.
78. Spark RF: *The Infertile Male: The Clinician's Guide to Diagnosis and Treatment.* New York, Plenum Medical Book Co, 1988.
79. Awadolla SG, Friedman CI, Schmidt G, et al: In vitro fertilization and embryo transfer as treatment for male factor infertility. *Fertil Steril* 1987; 47:807–811.
80. Amelar RD, Dubin L: Right varicocelectomy in selected infertile patients who have failed to improve after previous left varicocelectomy. *Fertil Steril* 1987; 47:833–837.
81. Saypol DC: Varicocele, in García C-R, Mastroianni L Jr, Amelar RD, et al (eds): *Current Therapy of Infertility 1984–1985.* Toronto, Canada, BC Decker Inc, 1984, pp 218–221.
82. Kursh ED: What is the incidence of varicocele in a fertile population? *Fertil Steril* 1987; 48:510–511.
83. Hudson RW: The endocrinology of varicoceles. *Fertil Steril* 1988; 49:199–208.
84. Dubin L, Amelar RD: Varicocelectomy: Twenty-five years of experience. *Int J Fertil* 1988; 33:226–235.
85. Dubin L, Amelar RD: Varcocelectomy: 986 cases in twelve year study. *Urology* 1977; 10:446–449.
86. Mehan DJ, Chehval MJ: Human chorionic gonadotropin in treatment of infertile man. *J Urol* 1982; 128:60–63.
87. Check JH: Improved semen quality in subfertile males with varicocele-associated oligospermia following treatment with clomiphene citrate. *Fertil Steril* 1980; 33:423–426.
88. Cockett ATK, Takihara H, Cosentino MJ: Varicocele. *Fertil Steril* 1984; 41:5–11.
89. Sherins RJ: Hypogonadotropic hypogonadism, in García C-R, Mastroianni L Jr, Amelar RD, et al (eds): *Current Therapy of Infertility 1984–1985.* Toronto, Canada, BC Decker Inc, 1984, pp 147–152.
90. Matsumoto AM, Karpas AE, Bremner WJ: Chronic human chorionic gona-

dotropin administration in normal men: Evidence that follicle-stimulating hormone is necessary for the maintenance of quantitatively normal spermatogenesis in man. *J Clin Endocrinol Metab* 1986; 62:1184–1192.

91. Burris AS, Rodbard HW, Winters SJ, et al: Gonadotropin therapy in men with isolated hypogonadotropin hypogonadism: Response to human chorionic gonadotropin is predicted by initial testicular size. *J Clin Endocrinol Metab* 1988; 66:1144–1151.

92. Shargil AA: Treatment of idiopathic hypogonadotropic hypogonadism in men with luteinizing hormone-releasing hormone: Comparison of treatment with daily injections and with the pulsatile infusion pump. *Fertil Steril* 1987; 47:492–501.

93. Aulitzky W, Frick J, Galvan G: Pulsatile luteinizing hormone-releasing hormone treatment of male hypogonadotropic hypogonadism. *Fertil Steril* 1988; 50:480–487.

94. Gross KM, Matsumoto AM, Bremner WJ: Differential control of luteinizing hormone and follicle-stimulating hormone secretion by luteinizing hormone-releasing hormone pulse frequency in man. *J Clin Endocrinol Metab* 1987; 64:675–680.

95. Spratt DI, Finkelstein JS, Butler JP, et al: Effects of increasing the frequency of low doses of gonadotropin-releasing hormone (GnRH) on gonadotropin secretion in GnRH-deficient men. *J Clin Endocrinol Metab* 1987; 64:1179–1186.

96. Veldhuis JD, Johnson ML, Dufau ML: Preferential release of bioactive luteinizing hormone in response to endogenous and low dose exogenous gonadotropin-releasing hormone pulses in man. *J Clin Endocrinol Metab* 1987; 64:1275–1282.

97. Crowley WF Jr: Hypogonadotropic hypogonadism with gonadotropin-releasing hormones, in García C-R, Mastroianni L Jr, Amelar RD, et al (eds): *Current Therapy of infertility-3.* Toronto, Canada, BC Decker Inc, 1988, pp 192–195.

98. Klingmüller D, Schweikert HU: Maintenance of spermatogenesis by intranasal administration of gonadotropin-releasing hormone in patients with hypothalamic hypogonadism. *J Clin Endocrinol Metab* 1985; 61:868–872.

99. Winters SJ, Troen P: Altered pulsatile secretion of luteinizing hormone in hypogonadal men with hyperprolactinaemia. *Clin Endocrinol (Oxf)* 1984; 21:257–263.

100. Sokol RZ, Steiner BS, Bustillo M, et al: A controlled comparison of the efficacy of clomiphene citrate in male infertility. *Fertil Steril* 1988; 49:865–870.

101. Buvat J, Ardaens K, Lemaire A, et al: Increased sperm count in 25 cases of idiopathic normogonadotropic oligospermia following treatment with tamoxifen. *Fertil Steril* 1983; 39:700–703.

102. AinMelk Y, Belisle S, Carmel M, et al: Tamoxifen citrate therapy in male infertility. *Fertil Steril* 1987; 48:113–117.

103. Paulson DF: Clomiphene citrate in management of male hypofertility: Predictors for treatment selection. *Fertil Steril* 1977; 28:1226–1229.

104. Amelar RD, Dubin L: Human chorionic gonadotropin therapy for idiopathic male infertility, in García C-R (ed): *Current Therapy of Infertility-3.* Toronto, Canada, BC Decker Inc, 1988, p 201.

105. Charny CW, Gordon JA: Testosterone rebound therapy: Neglected modality. *Fertil Steril* 1978; 29:64–68.

106. Brown JS: Effect of orally administered androgens on sperm motility. *Fertil Steril* 1975; 26:305–308.

107. Takihara H, Cosentino MJ, Cockett ATK: Effect of low-dose androgen and zinc sulfate on sperm motility and seminal zinc levels in infertile men. *Urology* 1983; 22:160–164.
108. Barkay J, Harpaz-Kerpel S, Ben-Ezra S, et al: Prostaglandin inhibitor effect of antiinflammatory drugs in therapy of male infertility. *Fertile Steril* 1984; 42:406–411.
109. Megory E, Zuckerman H, Shoham Z, et al: Infections and male fertility. *Obstet Gynecol Surv* 1987; 42:283–290.
110. Bronson RA: Current concepts on the relation of antisperm antibodies and infertility. *Semin Reprod Endocrinol* 1988; 6:363–368.
111. Tung K: Immunopathology and male infertility. *Hosp Pract [Off]* 1988; 191–206.
112. Alexander NJ, Sampson JH, Fulgham DL: Pregnancy rates in patients treated for antisperm antibodies with prednisone. *Int J Fertil* 1983; 28:63–67.
113. Shulman JF, Shulman S: Methylprednisolone treatment of immunologic infertility in male. *Fertil Steril* 1982; 38:591–599.
114. Bronson R, Cooper G, Rosenfeld D: Sperm antibodies: Their role in infertility. *Fertil Steril* 1984; 42:171–183.
115. Camitta BN, Storb R, Thomas ED: Aplastic anemia: Pathogenesis, diagnosis, treatment, and prognosis. *N Engl J Med* 1982; 306:712–718.
116. Webb OL, Laskarzewski PM, Glueck CJ: Severe depression of high-density lipoprotein cholesterol levels in weight lifters and body builders by self-administered exogenous testosterone and anabolic-androgenic steroids. *Metabolism* 1984; 33:971–975.
117. Hansten PD, Horn JR: *Drug Interactions: Clinical Significance of Drug-Drug Interactions,* ed 6. Philadelphia, Lea & Febiger, 1989.
118. MacAdams MR, White RH, Chipps BE: Reduction of serum testosterone levels during glucocorticoid therapy. *Ann Intern Med* 1986; 104:648–651.
119. Ross LS, Kandel GL, Prinz LM, et al: Clomiphene treatment of the idiopathic hypofertile male: High-dose, alternate-day therapy. *Fertil Steril* 1980; 33:618–623.
120. Saez JM, Forest MG: Kinetics of human chorionic gonadotropin-induced steroidogenic responses of human fetus, I: Plasma testosterone: Implication for human chorionic gonadotropin stimulation test. *J Clin Endocrinol Metab* 1979; 49:278–283.

Medical Management of Renal Stone Disease

Fredric L. Coe, M.D.

University of Chicago, Pritzker School of Medicine, Nephrology Program,
Chicago, Illinois

Joan Parks, M.B.A.

University of Chicago, Pritzker School of Medicine, Nephrology Program,
Chicago, Illinois

Readers of *Advances in Urology* know as much as any living group of doctors why kidney stones form and what treatments seem promising or useful, and for those who need reminding, new reviews abound.[1-4] What we add here are ways to circumvent problems of diagnosis, new findings concerning the efficacy of unproven remedies, and refinements to offset the naturally cumbersome character of certain treatments. We offer a new coat of varnish for well-prepared surfaces that may have weathered a bit these past few years, new luster for old wood.

Calcium Stones

Primary Hyperparathyroidism.—Routine limits of normal for serum calcium almost assure that you will overlook the subtle hypercalcemia we consider our most reliable clue to diagnosis (Fig 1). Our upper 95th percentile lies at the lines on Figure 1, and we use as our upper limits of normal 10.0 for women and 10.1 for men, and never have encountered a false-positive diagnosis. If we took 10.5 mg/dL as our upper limit, which is commonly done, we would not have sent half of these patients for surgical cure of their primary hyperparathyroidism. Some surely would have raised their blood calcium during medical treatment, or simply with time. Perhaps we might have called them examples of normocalcemic primary hyperparathyroidism[5, 6] unmasked by later events. Their very high urine calcium excretions (Fig 2) encourage confusion with the common familial or "idiopathic" hypercalciuria[7-9] usually treated with thiazide diuretic drugs. The thiazide diuretics raise the blood calcium level of patients with primary hyperparathyroidism,[10, 11] but also that of normal people.

Assay of parathyroid hormone levels never compensates for a failure to recognize hypercalcemia. Among patients who have proven hyperparathyroidism, the best assays (carboxy terminal antibody–based) are normal

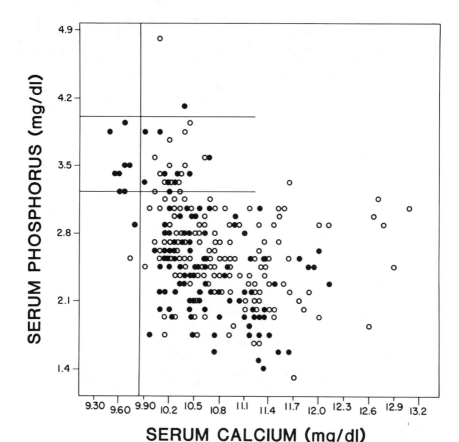

FIG 1.
Serum calcium and serum phosphorus values in men *(closed circles)* and women *(open circles)* with surgically proved hyperparathyroidism. A calcium level 2 SD above the normal mean is shown by the vertical line; one plus or minus 2 SD of the normal serum phosphorus level is shown by the two horizontal lines. (From Coe FL, Parks JH (eds): *Nephrolithiasis: Pathogenesis and Treatment.* Chicago, Year Book Medical Publishers, 1988. Used by permission.)

10% of the time, and so give a false-negative value that often (Fig 3); the worst assays (amino terminal–based) give false-negative values so often that they are useless. High levels of parathyroid hormone can occur in patients with familial hypercalciuria,[12] who do not benefit from surgery. One might say that for the diagnosis of hyperparathyroidism a low serum phosphorus level surpasses a high serum hormone level in accuracy (see Fig 1), as few patients lack this trait. At the very end of his career, one of our greatest teachers stressed the unique importance of hypercalcemia in distinguishing idiopathic hypercalciuria from primary hyperparathyroidism: "In fact the only distinguishing chemical feature is the normal serum calcium level as opposed to the high serum calcium level in hyperparathyroidism."[13]

Given the correct diagnosis, the main problems occur during surgery, especially in patients with parathyroid hyperplasia rather than a solitary parathyroid adenoma. Hyperplastic glands, which are recognized at surgery because at least two glands are enlarged, possess an unfortunate capacity to grow and re-create hyperparathyroidism.[14–16] Complete neck exploration, and a fine judgment regarding whether to leave a fragment of one gland in the neck or remove all glands and transplant tissue to a forearm, depend upon surgical experience, which is as difficult to judge as it is to acquire. Especially in community practice, such experience may be hard to find.

Normocalcemic Hypercalciuria.—A proper measurement of the daily urine calcium loss is the stumbling block that separates most doctors from a correct diagnosis. We collect three 24-hour urines while patients eat their regular diets, reasoning that decisions about a decade of treatment

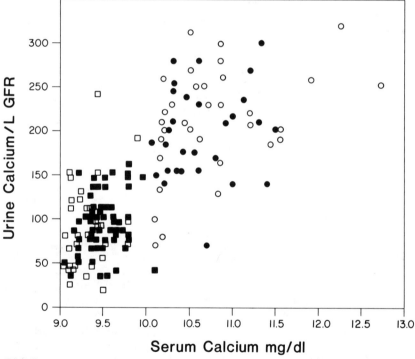

FIG 2.
Serum calcium (mg/dL) and urine calcium (mg/L GFR) in normal men *(closed squares)*, normal women *(open squares)*, and men *(closed circles)* and women *(open circles)* with primary hyperparathyroidism. (From Coe FL, Parks JH (eds): *Nephrolithiasis: Pathogenesis and Treatment.* Chicago, Year Book Medical Publishers, 1988. Used by permission.)

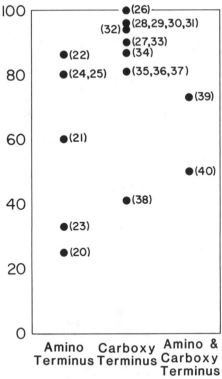

FIG 3.
Percent of amino terminus, carboxy terminus, and amino and carboxy terminus parathyroid hormone assay values elevated in surgically proven hyperparathyroidism. False-negative results occurred in 10% of the best carboxy terminus assays and in over 50% of the amino terminus assays. (From Coe FL, Parks JH (eds): *Nephrolithiasis: Pathogenesis and Treatment.* Chicago, Year Book Medical Publishers, 1988. Used by permission.)

warrant 3 days of effort, that we have most interest about urine excretions during the normal life of our patients and not during their use of a contrived diet, and that the financial expense of even a single stone passage episode can easily exceed the cost of measurements should one need an emergency room visit or a urological procedure. We compare the mean calcium excretion to normal means for each sex, using t-tests, and consider absolute excretion in milligrams, and excretion per gram of urine creatinine per liter of 24-hour creatinine clearance, or kilogram of body weight. We have published our normals,[17] and urge that centers accumulate their own local normal data.

We accept as hypercalciuria a mean differing from same-sex normals at the $P < .05$ level. Alternative diagnostic tactics include comparing individual urine values to normal means determined locally by an individual stone laboratory, or to conventional upper limits of normal, which traditionally have been 250 mg in women, 300 mg in men, and above 140 mg/g of urine creatinine in either sex. Once normocalcemic hypercalciuria is documented, a clinical exclusion of systemic diseases such as sarcoidosis, malignant tumors, rapidly progressive osteoporosis, Paget's disease, hyperthyroidism, glucocorticoid excess, and renal tubular acidosis exercises most doctors only a little bit, as most hypercalciuric stone formers are obviously fit people who have familial hypercalciuria. For our convenience, we will henceforth refer to the familial or idiopathic hypercalciuria as simply hypercalciuria. "Idiopathic hypercalciuria," the older term for this condition, seems inappropriate now that we know it is a hereditary disorder.

Thiazide diuretics lower urine calcium and prevent recurrent stones. They lower urine calcium by increasing distal nephron calcium reabsorption,[18] but their chronic use also may reduce intestinal calcium absorption; in seven patients we have studied using calcium balance, chlorthalidone reduced urine calcium more than calcium absorption (Fig 4), so calcium retention increased. Whether the increase benefits the skeleton, or even if it persists for more than the 3-month period we studied, both are unknown. Stone recurrence by control patients (Fig 5) exceeded that of treated patients in each of six prospective trials lasting at least 2 years, even

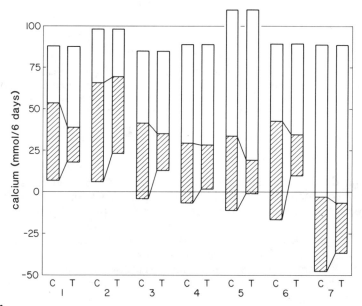

FIG 4.
Cumulative calcium balance for 6 days (mmol) in seven patients during control *(C)* and thiazide *(T)* period. The upper surface of each bar is the dietary intake, the open portion of the bar is fecal losses, and the cross-hatched portion is urine losses. Values above the zero line indicate positive balance-retention, below the line is the opposite. Chlorthalidone promotes mineral retention. (From Coe FL, Parks JH, Bushinsky DA, et al: *Kidney Int* 1988; 33:1140–1146. Used by permission.)

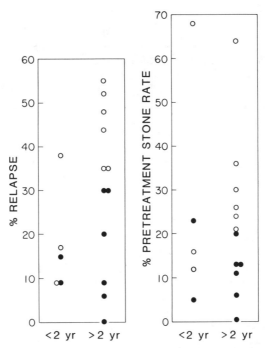

FIG 5.
Patients who relapsed on no treatment *(open circles)* and on thiazide treatment *(closed circles)*, followed for less than *(left side of panels)* or more than *(right side of panels)* 2 years. The left side of the figure shows the percentage of patients who relapsed and the right side shows the same patients with their treatment stone rates expressed as percent of pretreatment stone rates. (From Coe FL, Parks JH (eds): *Nephrolithiasis: Pathogenesis and Treatment.* Chicago, Year Book Medical Publishers, 1988. Used by permission.)

though different thiazide-type diuretics were used. Shorter trials did not show a consistent thiazide effect. We presume thiazide prevents recurrence by reducing urine calcium concentration and calcium oxalate supersaturation. Our usual dose is one third of the normal full adult dose for whatever specific agent we choose, and we measure urine calcium during treatment to assess the need for more. We have no particular reason to favor one agent over another, though our tendency is to use trichlormethiazide, 2 mg twice daily as starting treatment, as the pills are shaped like four-leaf clovers and have an attractive color.

A low-calcium diet also can lower urine calcium, and may be reasonable for some patients, but we have reservations about its safety.[19] When we fed normal people and hypercalciuric patients a very low-calcium diet (Fig 6), the patients excreted more calcium than did the normals and many excreted more than they ate. Admittedly, the diet period was short (9 days) and urine calcium may have returned to normal had we waited. While los-

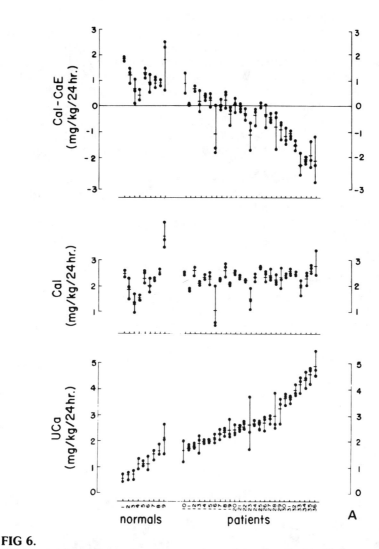

FIG 6.
Calcium intake and excretion in normal people and patients with hypercalciuria consuming a low-calcium diet. Mean calcium intakes of normal subjects and patients did not differ. Mean excretion rates during low-calcium diet *(lower panel)* of patients exceeded those of normals, and values of intake minus excretion *(Cal-CaE, top panel)* were negative in the majority of patients, but in no normals, showing that patients lost bone mineral in urine to a greater extent. (From Coe FL, Favus MJ, Sherwood LM, et al: Effects of low calcium diet on urine calcium excretion, parathyroid function and serum 1, 25 $(OH)_2 D_3$ levels in patients with idiopathic hypercalciuria and normal subjects. *Am J Med* 1982; 72:25–31. Used by permission.)

ing calcium in their urine in excess of diet intake, the patients maintained low serum parathyroid hormone levels (Fig 7) and did not display the normal fall in serum calcium concentration, as if their bone calcium loss into serum did not depend upon an increase in serum parathyroid hormone or a fall in blood calcium level. We believe their abnormal response to a low-calcium diet favors the theory that hypercalciuria frequently arises from excessive 1,25-dihydroxy vitamin D (calcitriol) production, as serum calcitriol levels were normal despite low parathyroid hormone, which should have lowered calcitriol, and higher than normal serum calcium level, which also should have lowered calcitriol levels of the patients below those of the normals.

Evidence for this theory includes a nearly universal finding of elevated serum calcitriol levels in hypercalciuric patients (Fig 8) along with the increased intestinal calcium absorption one would expect as a physiological consequence of calcitriol's effects upon intestinal cells. As well, the calcitriol levels of patients do not behave normally when dietary calcium is raised; after a brief fall, they rise, as if escaping from regulation.[20, 21] Serum calcitriol levels were normal in our patients during low-calcium diet intake, but serum parathyroid hormone was very low and serum calcium was above normal, and both factors should have suppressed calcitriol levels. Serum phosphorus levels were normal (not shown). Men given calcitriol in doses sufficient to raise urine, but not serum, calcium behave as our hypercalci-

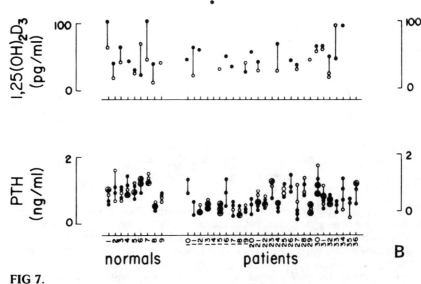

FIG 7.
Serum parathyroid hormone *(PTH)* and calcitriol in patients and normal subjects on their free-choice diets and a low-calcium diet. From Coe FL, Favus MJ, Sherwood LM, et al: Effects of low calcium diet on urine calcium excretion, parathyroid function and serum 1, 25 $(OH)_2$ D_3 levels in patients with idiopathic hypercalciuria and normal subjects. *Am J Med* 1982; 72:25–31. Used by permission.)

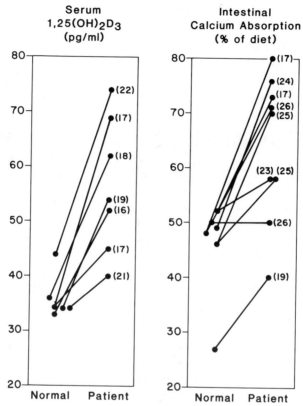

FIG 8.
Serum calcitriol levels and intestinal calcium absorption in normal subjects and in patients with familial hypercalciuria. (From Coe FL, Parks JH (eds): *Nephrolithiasis: Pathogenesis and Treatment.* Chicago, Year Book Medical Publishers, 1988. Used by permission.)

uric patients behaved when eating a very low-calcium diet (Fig 9); urine calcium remained too high, as in our patients, and calcium retention fell below normal.

Whether or not calcitriol proves the efficient cause of hypercalciuria, and whether or not all, most, or only some patients respond abnormally to a low-calcium diet, thiazide presently seems the more desirable treatment despite all of its natural drawbacks and inconveniences, and we favor using it as primary treatment. We recognize that our view is only one of many, and we have assumed our position fully aware that doctors always have been just as certain of their treatments as they have been wrong.

Hypocitraturia.—We prescribe potassium citrate along with thiazide not only to prevent arrhythmia and glucose intolerance, but also because hypokalemia reduces urine levels of citrate,[22] which normally attracts into a soluble salt nearly one half of urine calcium that could otherwise crystallize with oxalate or phosphate[23] to form stones. We also prescribe potas-

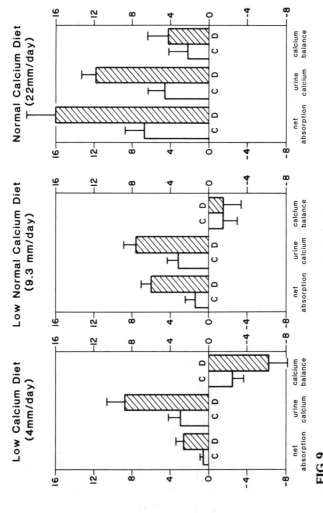

FIG 9.
Intestinal absorption, urine calcium, and calcium balance in normal men receiving calcitriol (cross-hatched bars) and in controls (open bars) at varying levels of calcium intake. (From Coe FL, Parks JH (eds): *Nephrolithiasis: Pathogenesis and Treatment.* Chicago, Year Book Medical Publishers, 1988. Used by permission.)

sium citrate for patients whose urine citrate levels are low from diseases, such as renal tubular acidosis[24] or intestinal malabsorption, and for the rather large group of patients whose urine citrate levels are low for reasons we do not understand.

Patients in this last group have normal blood citrate levels and filter normal amounts of citrate into their renal tubules, but their tubules reabsorb citrate in excess of normal and leave only a little for urine excretion. Although idiopathic hypocitraturia occurs in both sexes, females exhibit it more dramatically and consistently. Women who form calcium oxalate stones (Fig 10) excrete so much less citrate than do normal women that their low urine citrate level elevates calcium oxalate supersaturation as much as does their hypercalciuria.[25] Normal men excrete urine with calcium and citrate levels matching those of stone-forming women, and we suspect that this accounts for the extreme male susceptibility to stone disease,[25] which most place at fivefold above that of women. Men who form stones excrete more calcium and water than do normal men but about the same amount of citrate, so even though they do not exhibit marked hypocitraturia, their urine ratio of citrate to calcium is low and their urine levels of free calcium ion are high.

We could prescribe citrate or bicarbonate as pills or capsules of the sodium salt and diminish complaints from dissatisfied patients who dislike the flavor of the effervescent potassium citrate preparations that must be taken dissolved in water, and resent the expensive and bothersome daily alternative of six or eight very large wax capsules. We struggle with potassium

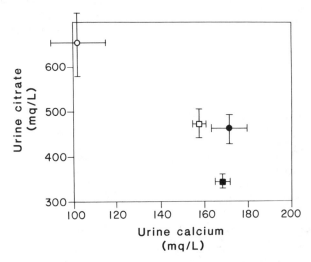

FIG 10.
Urine citrate vs. calcium concentration (± SEM) in women *(open symbols)* and men *(closed symbols)* with *(square)* and without *(circles)* calcium oxalate nephrolithiasis. (From Parks JH, Coe FL: *Kidney Int* 1986; 30:85–90. Used by permission.)

salts even for patients who are not hypercalciuric and do not use thiazide diuretics because sodium loading raises urine calcium excretion[26] and blood pressure. We use 25 mEq of alkali twice daily and measure urine citrate to determine efficacy.

Hyperoxaluria.—We measure oxalate in the same three urines that we obtain for detecting hypercalciuria, and diagnose hyperoxaluria when the mean of three oxalate excretion measurements exceeds the mean for same-sex normals at the level of $P < .05$. We also cast a cold eye on sporadic high values, above 40 mg daily, because diet oxalate influences urine oxalate excretion and some patients are impetuous and disorderly about their food, gorging on spinach one day, egg salad the next. We have ascribed all sporadic hyperoxaluria and most instances of consistent hyperoxaluria to diet, as most patients do not suffer from intestinal diseases that cause malabsorption,[27] excrete oxalate at only modestly high rates of 50 to 60 mg daily (well below the values found in hereditary forms of primary hyperoxaluria[28]) and respond to an improved diet with gratifying abatement of their hyperoxaluria. We offer our patients a conventional diet list that can be found anywhere[29] and exhort them to embrace it as their gospel and to perfect themselves and find salvation through its teachings.

Most of the remaining patients are hyperoxaluric because their small intestines absorb their food incompletely and permit bile salts, medium chain length fatty acids, and other digestive products that normally would be absorbed to escape into the colon. They damage the lining of the colon and oxalate, along with other innocuous molecules like amino acids, urea, and glucose, leak into the blood from the colon lumen simply because the kidneys constantly filter and secrete oxalate out of the blood and keep its concentration there very low compared to its levels in intestinal fluids. When the kidneys fail, blood oxalate rises to levels usual in urine, 200 to 300 µM, and blood supersaturates with respect to calcium oxalate, which can crystallize in blood vessel walls, kidneys, the heart, the testicles, joint fluid, and almost everywhere else.[30] When they are normal, they excrete all the oxalate from metabolism and diet each day, even if they damage themselves in the process. Usual levels of urine oxalate in intestinal malabsorption range from normal to up to 200 or 250 mg daily, the highest values being far above those of most routine dietary hyperoxaluria, but the diagnosis of an enteric cause for oxaluria rests on clinical assessment of the bowel disease, not on the urine oxalate level.

Although diminishing dietary fat and oxalate can alleviate enteric hyperoxaluria, intestinal malabsorption restricts the nutrition of many patients so greatly that they cannot safely relinquish whole categories of foods, especially those high in calories. Oral supplements of calcium can precipitate food oxalate as the calcium oxalate salt, which cannot be absorbed, provided calcium is taken in a dose of 1 to 3 g with meals. Cholestyramine binds oxalate[31] as well as the bile salts and unabsorbed fatty acids that would damage the colon lining, and reduces hyperoxaluria when taken as 1 to 4 g with each meal.[32] Sometimes cholestyramine causes abdominal pain and even partial intestinal obstruction, or worsens diarrhea. Because it binds vitamin K, prothrombin time may increase. Many patients dislike its flavor or texture. We always endeavor to use all four treatments together, each one at a level which enables the ensemble to achieve sufficient results with minimum travail. Usually, diet changes prove impractical, calcium supplements increase to 2 or 3 g with each meal, and cholestyramine increases to its maximum of 4 g four times daily and yet high urine oxalate persists.

Because of reduced intestinal bicarbonate reabsorption, alkaline diarrhea occurs in many patients and causes metabolic acidosis that reduces urine citrate excretion. Oral alkali supplements compensate for stool alkali losses, and are best given as a sodium salt, even as simple 10-grain sodium bicarbonate tablets, at a total dose of 40 to 60 mEq of base in three divided doses each day. Patients with ileostomy never develop enteric hyperoxaluria, but form stones from dehydration and low urine citrate and pH and benefit from oral alkali.

Primary hyperoxaluria occurs from hereditary enzyme deficiencies[28] and has no specific treatment. Oral pyridoxine, 10 to up to 1,000 mg daily in graduated doses may benefit some; we have tried it, using an ascending dosage schedule guided by repeated urine measurements, and never have observed a fall in oxalate excretion. Others[32] have. Raising urine citrate may benefit these patients.

Hyperuricosuria.—When we[33] first reported that up to 25% of calcium oxalate stone-formers excreted more uric acid than did normals of the same sex and age distribution, and responded to allopurinol by reducing their new stone formation rates, doctors generally were surprised, and scientists who worked then on stone disease were dubious and skeptical. By now our observation has achieved the distinction of a perfect confirmation, most recently in a prospective trial of allopurinol vs. placebo in calcium stone-formers[34] who had no cause for stones except hyperuricosuria (Fig 11). Dietary excess of purine causes the hyperuricosuria, an excessive eating of beef, chicken, and fish in place of grains and starches[35] that seems a perfectly American gourmandism, so diet alteration alone can be an ample treatment. We diagnose hyperuricosuria by *t*-tests of the mean of three measurements against same-sex normals, just as for hypercalciuria, and we respond to sporadic high values, above 800 mg daily in men and 750 mg in women, by offering dietary advice. Some patients, mostly men, will not relinquish their rich diets despite recurrent stones and our determined appeals to the rational sides of their natures, compelling us to offer allopurinol.

Doctors exhibit a surprising desire to know why therapies succeed and a reluctance to embrace and use what is mysterious, and because they so desire explanation we have sought the true reason why uric acid and calcium stones are linked. One theory holds that uric acid crystals offer a surface so similar to calcium oxalate that ions in solution cannot tell the two apart and grow as well on the one as on the other, so-called heterogeneous nucleation.[36] Another holds that adsorption of amino acids or other urine molecules on uric acid crystals makes their surfaces ideal starting

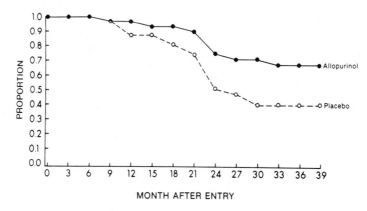

MONTH AFTER ENTRY

Life-Table Plot Showing Proportion of Patients without
Calculous Events during Treatment with Allopurinol or Placebo.

FIG 11.
Life table plot showing proportion of patients without calculous events during treatment with allopurinol or placebo. (From Ettinger B, Tang A, and Citron JT: *N Engl J Med* 1986; 315:1386–1389. Used by permission.)

points for calcium oxalate crystals.[37] Both theories are supported by the finding of some uric acid in stones of about 10% to 12% of calcium oxalate stone-formers, a subgroup that also includes a high fraction of patients who are prone to hyperuricosuria. Yet another theory holds that uric acid crystals adsorb crystallization inhibitors and deprive the kidneys of a precious defense. Whichsoever proves correct, if any does, the facts of treatment will remain unaltered.

Abnormal Urine pH.—Our kidneys control urine pH by regulating bicarbonate reabsorption and proton excretion,[38] and do so mainly to balance daily acid excretion against daily proton load from diet and metabolism. Ammonia excretion confers upon them a limited freedom, since protons excreted with ammonia, as ammonium ions, do not require that urine pH be much below that of blood; put another way, ammonium ion regulation can stand in place of change in urine pH at a constant net acid excretion.

Certainly, this freedom has evolved to protect against otherwise inevitable stones. Were ammonium excretion set at a low fixed level, pH would fall whenever we ate meat, and uric acid crystals would form and either promote calcium stones or uric acid stones. The pK for the first proton dissociation off uric acid is 5.3 in urine, and dihydrogen urate solubility in urine is only 98 mg/L.[39] At an average daily pH of 5.3, we could not safely excrete normal amounts of uric acid (500 to 600 mg) in even 2 L of urine; but at the normal average pH of 6, we can excrete 800 mg daily in 1 L. Among hyperuricosuric calcium oxalate stone-formers we have found traces of an evolutionary limitation, in that many form mixed calcium uric acid stones and have average urine pH values of 5.6.[40] They do not fully adapt ammonium production to balance proton excretion at a pH of 6. When we encounter low average pH, we advise alkali supplements, though this tactic never has been formally tested for efficacy in calcium stone-formers.

At the other extreme, there exist patients whose urine pH is abnormally high, either because of renal tubular acidosis, alkali excess, or diets that impose an unusually low proton load. A urine pH much above 6.5 raises the urine levels of trivalent phosphate anion and carbonate, leading to calcium phosphate and calcium carbonate stones.[38] Diet and alkali excess we treat in a simple manner. Renal tubular acidosis usually is secondary to familial hypercalciuria[41] with nephrocalcinosis, and we treat patients with thiazide. Rare patients who have hereditary distal renal tubular acidosis and hypercalciuria secondary to metabolic acidosis[42] we treat with alkali.

Uric Acid Stones

We have already disclosed the central mystery; as urine pH falls below 6.0 and nears the pK for the first proton of uric acid, more and more of the urine uric acid becomes converted into dihydrogen urate, which is insoluble and forms stones. Calculate the urine concentration of undissociated uric acid (dihydrogen urate) from our nomogram (Fig 12) using total uric acid concentration and pH from each of the three 24-hour samples you will have obtained during your evaluation of your patient, compare each value to the solubility of 98 mg/L, and offer your patient about 25 mEq of alkali twice daily if supersaturation is modest and 50 mEq twice daily if it is severe. Recheck the urine in a few weeks and readjust. If you have a perfectionistic streak, ask patients to check the pH of each voiding for a time and adjust timing to achieve an ideal of therapeutic intervention, a value of 6 each time. If you do this, you will need allopurinol only rarely, when daily uric acid excretion exceeds 1,000 mg, urine pH simply will not rise to 6.0, or a patient lacks reliability or perhaps cannot be bothered with several treatments each day.

Cystinuria

Maybe more than most diseases, this one calls to mind that we require a knowledge of principles and a knowledge of particulars, that lacking one we become useless, and lacking the other ignorant practitioners of remedies. Urine can dissolve cystine in only modest amounts (Fig 13) and those rare people who lack the renal cell transporters to reabsorb cystine properly lose enough in the urine to form stones. That other amino acids share transporters with cystine and are lost, that the hereditary disorders of renal transporters are various and some also affect intestinal cell amino transport, and that the exact fate of cystine remains partly mysterious, all can enlighten us, but we prefer to omit these details not because we endorse

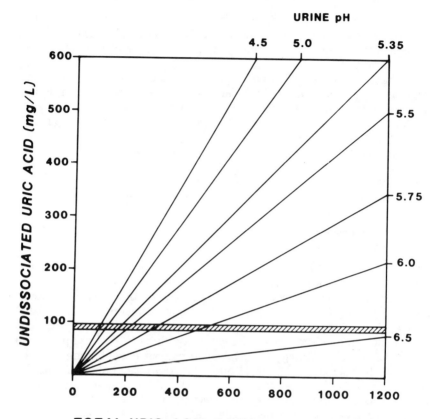

URINE pH

FIG 12.
Nomogram showing undissociated uric acid concentration at values of urine pH and total uric acid concentration. The solubility limit for uric acid is shown by *cross-hatched bars* (96 ± 2 mg/L). (From Coe FL: *Kidney Int* 1983; 24:392–403. Used by permission.)

unenlightenment, but because they have almost no use for clinical work.

Howsoever urine cystine becomes elevated, stones are prevented by greater urine volume for dilution and by drugs that reduce cystine concentration. To calculate the amount of urine a patient needs, simply divide the daily urine cystine excretion by the mean cystine solubility (Fig 14). We believe that kidneys excrete cystine constantly by day and night, and encourage nocturia that eventually discourages most patients who otherwise might need no other treatment than water, even though we have no proof that nocturia is essential.

For those whom water cannot treat, we use drugs that reduce urine cystine concentration by binding to cysteine more strongly than cysteine can bind to itself to dimerize into cystine. The best known agent is D-penicil-

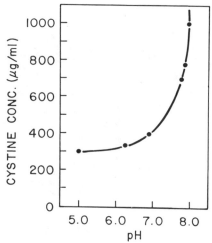

FIG 13.
The solubility of cystine in relation to urinary pH. (From Dent CE, Senior B: *Br J Urol* 1955; 27:317. Used by permission.)

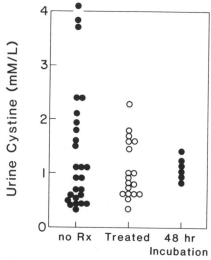

FIG 14.
Urine concentrations of cystine (mM/L) in men and women with untreated cysti-nuria, cystinuria treated with D-penicillamine, and 48-hour incubation with 10 mg/mL of cystine showing range of urine cystine solubility. (From Coe FL, Parks JH (eds): *Nephrolithiasis: Pathogenesis and Treatment.* Chicago, Year Book Medical Publishers, 1988. Used by permission.)

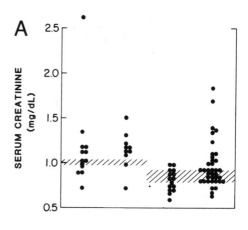

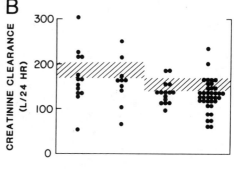

FIG 15.
Serum creatinine levels (mg/dL, **A**), creatinine clearance (L/24 hours, **B**), and urine calcium levels (mg/g of creatinine, **C**) in men and women with pure and mixed struvite stones. The *bars* represent means ± 1 SD of normal subjects studied in the same laboratory. (From Kristensen C, Parks JH, Lindheimer M, et al: *Kidney Int* 1987; 32:749–753. Used by permission.)

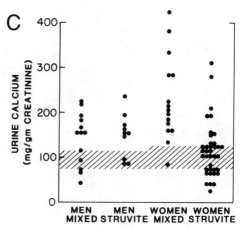

lamine, used as 1 to 2 g daily. N-acetyl D-penicillamine—marketed in the United States as Mucomist and not approved for oral use in cystine stone prevention—is used orally for the treatment of acetaminophen toxicity and can act exactly as D-penicillamine, which it closely resembles. Thiopronin (Thiola) now is available for routine use in the United States as 100-mg tablets.

The drugs all share a sulfhydryl side group, which reacts with the corresponding group on cysteine to form a soluble mixed disulfide, and drugs of this type can cause serious side effects of rash, fever, nausea, pancytopenia, arthritis, a systemic lupus-like syndrome, and nephrotic syndrome; thiopronin seems less likely to cause these reactions. Loss of taste and smell may occur with penicillamine and may respond to zinc supplements. Because they are dangerous, we always hope to avoid these drugs, or to use them only from time to time.

Struvite Stones

Most of our urologist friends seem to know much more than we do about these terrible stones, about the versatile and hardy bacteria that produce them and how perilous the future of any unfortuante kidney they invade, and certainly about the imagination and dexterity one must exercise for their removal. But we who do nothing surgical, who mostly observe, know

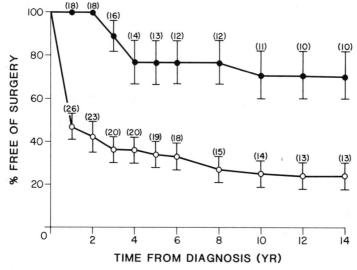

FIG 16.
Occurrence of urinary tract surgery in 75 patients with struvite nephrolithiasis whose first symptom was *(closed circles)* and was not *(open circles)* stone passage. (From Kristensen C, Parks JH, Lindheimer M, et al: *Kidney Int* 1987; 32:749–753. Used by permission.)

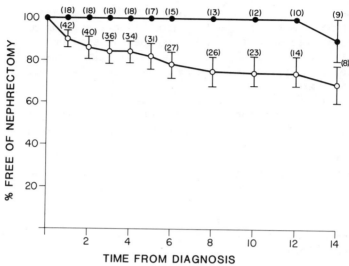

FIG 17.
Occurrence of nephrectomy in 75 patients wtih struvite nephrolithiasis whose first symptom was *(closed circles)* and was not *(open circles)* stone passage. (From Kristensen C, Parks JH, Lindheimer M, et al: *Kidney Int* 1987; 32:749–753. Used by permission.)

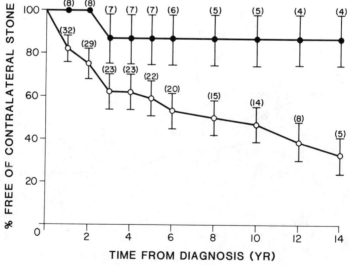

FIG 18.
Development of a contralateral stone in 50 patients wtih unilateral struvite nephrolithiasis whose first symptom was *(closed circles)* and was not *(open circles)* stone passage. (From Kristensen C, Parks JH, Lindheimer M, et al: *Kidney Int* 1987; 32:749–753. Used by permission.)

a few details that could interest men of action.[43] Some patients form stru- vite stones that also contain calcium oxalate, and these "mixed" stone- formers usually have genetic hypercalciuria (Fig 15) as well as urinary in- fection, whereas the patients whose struvite stones are "pure" (free of cal- cium oxalate) usually do not. Women with pure stones tend to have re- duced creatinine clearance, unlike the other groups. If stones present with ← passage, they are likely to be mixed, and to carry much less risk of urinary ← tract surgery (Fig 16), eventual nephrectomy (Fig 17), or contralateral ← stone development (Fig 18). We presume that pure struvite stones reflect only urinary infection, and that mixed stones reflect the combination of metabolic stones and superimposed infection.

Most new treatments are surgical, related to extracorporeal shock wave lithotripsy, percutaneous nephrolithotomy, and new endoureteral instru- ments; we can barely pronounce some of these treatments, and surely do not write about them. Acetohydroxamic acid falls within our medical pur- view. This inhibitor of bacterial urease slows stone growth,[44] but side ef- fects force 20% of patients to stop using it. The drug is teratogenic, and may cause germ cell or somatic cell gene mutations. We consider the drug a very minor contribution to treatment, because of its side effects, and have almost no clinical experience with it despite our large number of stru- vite stone patients, a fact that may say more about the true situation than does citing references or research concerning mechanisms of drug action.

References

1. Coe FL, Parks JH: Pathophysiology of kidney stones and strategies for treat- ment. *Hosp Pract [Off]* 1988; 23:185–207.
2. Smith LH: The medical aspects of urolithiasis: An overview. *J Urol* 1989; 141:707–710.
3. Drach GW: Surgical overview of urolithiasis. *J Urol* 1989; 141:711–713.
4. Pak CYC: Role of medical prevention. *J Urol* 1989; 141:798–801.
5. Johnson RD, Conn JW: Hyperparathyroidism with a prolonged period of nor- mocalcemia. *JAMA* 1969; 210:2063–2066.
6. Yendt ER, Gagne RJA: Detection of primary hyperparathyroidism, with special reference to its occurrence in hypercalciuric females with "normal" or border- line serum calcium. *Can Med Assoc J* 1968; 98:331–336.
7. Robertson WG, Morgan DB: The distribution of urinary calcium excretions in normal persons and stone-formers. *Clin Chim Acta* 1972; 37:503.
8. Sutton RAL: Disorders of renal calcium excretion. *Kidney Int* 1983; 23:665–673.
9. Bordier P, Ryck A, Guerio J, et al: On the pathogenesis of so-called idiopathic hypercalciuria. *Am J Med* 1977; 63:398–409.
10. Duarte DG, Winnacker JL, Becker KL, et al: Thiazide-induced hypercalcemia. *N Engl J Med* 1971; 284:828–830.
11. Parfitt AM: Thiazide-induced hypercalcemia in vitamin D-treated hypoparathy- roidism. *Ann Intern Med* 1972; 77:557–563.
12. Pak CYC, Ohata M, Lawrence EC, et al: The hypercalciurias: Causes, par- athyroid functions and diagnostic criteria. *J Clin Invest* 1974; 54:387–400.

13. Henneman PH, Benedict P, Forbes AP, et al: Idiopathic hypercalciuria. *N Engl J Med* 1958; 259:802–807.
14. Wells SA, Ellis GJ, Gunnells JC, et al: Parathyroid autotransplantation in primary parathyroid hyperplasia. *N Engl J Med* 1976; 295:57–62.
15. Brennan MF, Brown EM, Marx SJ, et al: Recurrent hyperparathyroidism from an autotransplanted parathyroid adenoma. *N Engl J Med* 1978; 299:1057–1059.
16. Maschio G, Vecchioni R, Tessitore N: Recurrence of autonomous hyperparathyroidism in calcium nephrolithiasis. *Am J Med* 1980; 69:607–609.
17. Coe FL, Parks JH: Clinical approach, in Coe FL, Parks JH (eds): *Nephrolithiasis: Pathogenesis and Treatment,* ed 2. Chicago, Year Book Medical Publishers, 1988, p 34.
18. Costanzo LS: Localization of diuretic action in microperfused rat distal tubules: Ca and NA transport. *Am J Physiol* 1985; 248:F527–535.
19. Coe FL, Favus MJ, Sherwood LM, et al: Effects of low calcium diet on urine calcium excretion, parathyroid function and serum 1,25 $(OH)_2D_3$ levels in patients with idiopathic hypercalciuria and normal subjects. *Am J Med* 1982; 72:25–32.
20. Adams ND, Gray RW, Lemann J Jr: The effects of oral $CaCo_3$ loading and dietary calcium deprivation on plasma 1,25-dihydroxyvitamin D concentration in healthy adults. *J Clin Endocrinol Metab* 1979; 148:1008–1016.
21. Maierhofer WJ, Lemann J Jr, Gray RW, et al: Dietary calcium and serum 1,25-$(OH)_2$-vitamin D concentrations as determinants of calcium balance in healthy men. *Kidney Int* 1984; 26:752–759.
22. Nicar MJ, Peterson R, Pak CYC: Use of potassium citrate as potassium supplement during thiazide therapy of calcium nephrolithiasis. *J Urol* 1984; 131:430–433.
23. Meyer JL: Formation constants for interaction of citrate with calcium and magnesium ions. *Anal Biochem* 1974; 62:295–300.
24. Dedmon RE, Wrong O: The excretion of organic anion in renal tubular acidosis with particular reference to citrate. *Clin Sci* 1962; 22:19–32.
25. Parks JH, Coe FL: A urinary-calcium citrate index for the evaluation of nephrolithiasis. *Kidney Int* 1986; 30:85–90.
26. Muldowney FP, Freaney R, Moloney MF: Importance of dietary sodium in the hypercalciuric syndrome. *Kidney Int* 1982; 22:292–296.
27. Smith LH, Fromm H, Hoffman AF: Acquired hyperoxaluria, nephrolithiasis and intestinal disease. *N Engl J Med* 1972; 286:1371.
28. Williams HE, Smith LH Jr: Primary hyperoxaluria, in Stanbury JB, Wyngaarden JB, Fredrickson DS (eds): *The Metabolic Basis of Inherited Disease,* ed 5. New York, McGraw-Hill Book Co, 1983, pp 204–288.
29. Coe FL, Parks JH: Hyperoxaluric states, in Coe FL, Parks JH (eds): *Nephrolithiasis: Pathogenesis and Treatment,* ed 2. Chicago, Year Book Medical Publishers, 1988, pp 198–200.
30. Worcester EM, Nakagawa Y, Bushinsky DA, et al: Evidence that serum calcium oxalate supersaturation is a consequence of oxalate retention in patients with chronic renal failure. *J Clin Invest* 1986; 77:1888–1896.
31. Coe FL, Parks JH: Hyperoxaluric states, in Coe FL, Parks JH (eds): *Nephrolithiasis: Pathogenesis and Treatment,* ed 2. Chicago, Year Book Medical Publishers, 1988, pp 197–200.
32. Yendt ER, Cohanim M: Response to physiologic dose of pyridoxine in type 1 primary hyperoxaluria. *N Engl J Med* 1985; 312:953–957.

33. Coe FL, Raisen L: Allopurinol treatment of uric-acid disorders in calcium-stone formers. *Lancet* 1973; 1:129.
34. Ettinger B, Tang A, Citron JT, et al: Randomized trial of allopurinol in the prevention of calcium oxalate calculi. *N Engl J Med* 1986; 315:1386–1389.
35. Kavalich AG, Moran E, Coe FL: Dietary purine consumption by hyperuricosuric calcium oxalate kidney stone formers and normal subjects. *J Chronic Dis* 1976; 29:745.
36. Deganello S, Coe FL: Epitaxy between uric acid and whewellite: Experimental verification. *Neues Jahrbuch Minerologia* 1983; 6:270–276.
37. Finlayson B, DuBois L: Adsorption of heparin on sodium acid urate. *Clin Chim Acta* 1978; 84:203–206.
38. Coe FL, Parks JH: Calcium phosphate stones and renal tubular acidosis, in Coe FL, Parks JH (eds): *Nephrolithiasis: Pathogenesis and Treatment,* ed 2. Chicago, Year Book Medical Publishers, 1988, pp 149–157.
39. Coe FL, Strauss AL, Tembe V, et al: Uric acid saturation in calcium nephrolithiasis. *Kidney Int* 1980; 17:662–668.
40. Coe FL: Uric acid and calcium oxalate nephrolithiasis. *Kidney Int* 1983; 24:392–403.
41. Stinebaugh BJ, Schloeder FX, Tam SC, et al: Pathogenesis of distal renal tubular acidosis. *Kidney Int* 1981; 19:1–7.
42. Coe FL, Parks JH: Stone disease in hereditary distal renal tubular acidosis. *Ann Intern Med* 1980; 93:60–61.
43. Kristensen C, Parks JH, Lindheimer M, et al: Reduced glomerular filtration rate and hypercalciuria in primary struvite nephrolithiasis. *Kidney Int* 1987; 32:749–753.
44. Griffith DP: Infection-induced renal calculi. *Kidney Int* 1982; 21:422–430.

The Pathophysiology of Incontinence in the Elderly

Pat D. O'Donnell, M.D.

Professor, Department of Urology, University of Arkansas for Medical Sciences, College of Medicine, Department of Urology, Director, Arkansas Center for Incontinence, Chief, Little Rock Veterans Administration Medical Center, Little Rock, Arkansas

Urinary incontinence is a serious problem of the elderly and its economic, social, and medical impact on their medical care is immense. At the present time, approximately 38 million Americans are over 60 years of age.[1] Of these individuals who live independently, approximately 38% of women and 19% of men experience urinary incontinence.[2] Of elderly people in chronic care facilities, approximately 55% experience urinary incontinence.[3] At the present time, over 1.5 million elderly people are in nursing homes in the United States.[1] The total direct health care cost of urinary incontinence in this country in 1987 was approximately $10.3 billion.[1] The annual cost of management of urinary incontinence in these patients is more than the combined annual cost of coronary artery bypass surgery and renal dialysis.[4] Although the medical, economic, and social impact of urinary incontinence in the elderly is significant, many aspects of the etiology of incontinence in this group remain unclear and clinical investigation in this area has been limited.

An important initial step in the approach to management of urinary incontinence in the elderly has been physician and patient awareness of its prevalence and the many ways in which it affects this population. Much effort has been made during recent years to increase awareness of the problem among physicians and patients. For example, the National Institutes of Health sponsored the first Consensus Development Conference on Urinary Incontinence during 1988, which brought together clinicians and investigators from multiple clinical and research areas involved in the management of health care problems related to urinary incontinence. This program and others have helped to identify some of the clinical problems related to this disorder, define current treatment options, and outline research needs for the future. Organizations such as the Simon Foundation have dedicated their efforts to awareness and management issues related to urinary incontinence. Help for Incontinent People is a national organization dedicated to helping patients understand the problems of incontinence and the treatment options available.

Reprinted from *Advances in Urology,*® vol. 4.
Copyright 1991, Mosby–Year Book, Inc.

Clinical investigation into the problem of urinary incontinence in the elderly has been relatively recent, with most of the work being done in the last half of this century. In 1948, Wilson applied cystometric evaluation to elderly patients with this disorder.[5] He found that during filling cystometry, involuntary detrusor contractions were common in elderly incontinent patients.

This finding was duplicated subsequently by a number of other investigators.[6, 7] Unstable activity of the bladder in these patients is now considered to be a major factor in the etiology of incontinence.

Based on the clinical evaluation and treatment of elderly patients, an attempt has been made to classify incontinent patients into broad categories. Brocklehurst concluded that it is important to differentiate between transient and established incontinence.[8] He found that, for many reasons, elderly people may have a phase of urinary incontinence that often will resolve spontaneously or following treatment of an underlying contributing disorder. He called this transient urinary incontinence. Other patients have incontinence that persists even when their general condition is optimal; this is considered to represent established urinary incontinence.

Transient Incontinence

Acute medical problems in the elderly may result in transient episodes of urinary incontinence. This may occur following pneumonia, myocardial infarction, and other types of acute medical disorders. Less severe disorders, such as constipation or fecal impaction, may result in transient incontinence. The etiology of incontinence in patients with fecal impaction is unclear, but it is thought to be a type of overflow incontinence resulting from reflex inhibition of the bladder most likely produced by rectal stimulation.[9, 10] Acute inflammatory conditions of the lower urinary tract also may precipitate urinary incontinence.[11] The relationship of bacteriuria and pyuria to urinary incontinence is uncertain,[12, 13] but the presence of bacteriuria is generally thought to precipitate the problem in elderly people. In some cases, patients who already have established incontinence may develop medical problems that can cause a transient increase in its severity.

Established Incontinence

Established incontinence in elderly people usually occurs over a long period of time and is present even when the patient's general condition is stable. Urinary incontinence in these patients is often associated with functional mental disabilities and is commonly seen in patients who have dementia or focal neurological impairments following a stroke.[7] It also has been associated with functional physical disabilities and appears to increase in severity as physical activity diminishes.[7, 14,15] In addition, there appears to be a higher incidence of incontinence with increasing age that may be due to multiple factors, such as medications, that affect bladder function.[16, 17]

The clinical observations that associate the disorder with functional disabilities suggest that urinary incontinence in the elderly is related to a general deterioration of the central nervous system as well as of the general physical condition of the individual. This concept is further supported by the association of urinary incontinence in the elderly with a poor prognosis for long-term survival.[17, 18] The decrease in long-term survival may be related to conditions such as dementia, poor mobility, and poor physical health; incontinence is probably not a risk factor in its own right.[17]

While deterioration in mental and physical function has been found to be prevalent in incontinent patients, these trends are sometimes difficult to interpret in terms of the pathophysiology of incontinence by the clinician who is working with individual patients. For example, it is common for a clinician to observe severely demented patients who void voluntarily without incontinence. In addition, many stroke patients with severe physical and mental impairment void voluntarily. Finally, many bedridden male patients routinely void voluntarily into a urinal and rarely have an incontinence accident. Therefore, while ambulatory status appears to be a factor in urinary incontinence, it is not always important. These observations are difficult to explain in terms of our current understanding of the role of the central nervous system in the etiology of this disorder. Many important clinical characteristics are well recognized by daily caregivers of elderly patients, but their exact significance to the pathophysiology of incontinence has not been appreciated.

Incontinence Assessment

Examination of incontinence characteristics in elderly people requires accurate measurement of these events. The first step in the evaluation of incontinence or the implementation of a treatment plan is to assess accurately the severity of the clinical problem, which can be difficult to accomplish in the elderly. One of the most commonly used methods of assessment is a urinary diary. Because this method relies on the record-keeping capabilities of elderly patients, who are subject to varying degrees of cortical impairment, its accuracy may be questionable. Despite this shortcoming, however, the urinary diary has proved to be reliable in the assessment of incontinence severity in selected elderly community-dwelling patients.[18] Assessment is especially difficult in chronic care patients, who have a higher incidence of cortical impairment than do those who live in the community; self-reporting is not a reliable method of measuring incontinence in these individuals. Questionnaires and urinary diaries kept by elderly inpatients fail to yield reliable incontinence information.[19] Periodic "wet checks" performed by the nursing staff at fixed time intervals are commonly employed in this population. While this is a reasonably accurate detection method, it has some drawbacks. The optimal time interval between checks is unclear; every 2 to 4 hours is common practice. Chronic care nursing staff often have difficulty maintaining a constant interval between checks, and patients frequently complain about the intrusiveness of the procedure, especially when they are dry at the time of the check. Finally, this assessment technique applies a fixed schedule of measurement to events that have widely varying intervals of occurrence. Frequency data obtained using an electronic detection technique have shown that 56% of incontinence episodes in severely incontinent patients occur at intervals of 2 hours or less.[20]

Urodynamic Evaluation of Incontinence

Involuntary detrusor contraction during filling cystometry is the most common urodynamic finding in incontinent elderly patients.[21-25] Although detrusor instability is often referred to as a cause of incontinence in the elderly, it may be more appropriately considered to be a urodynamic finding associated with the disorder. Uninhibited detrusor contractions have been seen in 32% of elderly continent subjects compared to 50% of elderly incontinent sybjects.[25] The relationship of involuntary detrusor contractions during filling cystometry to the occurrence of urinary incontinence events currently is unclear, although there does seem to be a significantly higher incidence of incontinence in patients with this instability. Other aspects of filling cystometry that appear to be important are bladder capacity, sensation of fullness, and length of time the impending contraction is perceived by the patient before it actually occurs.

One of the problems with urodynamic assessment of the elderly is determining the presence of outflow obstruction. A pressure-flow study is commonly used to evaluate this possibility; however, it is sometimes difficult to assess due to the involuntary detrusor contractions that occur in the presence of the filling catheter used during cystometry. A microtip catheter alleviates this complication, since it results in minimal urethral obstruction and provides information on the maximum detrusor pressure during bladder contraction. Another difficulty with the pressure-flow study is that elderly patients often are unable to initiate voiding voluntarily. Obstruction of the bladder outlet is associated with detrusor instability.[26] Symptoms of detrusor compensation with obstruction, such as urgency, frequency, nocturia, and incontinence, are very similar to those provoked by central neural lesions. Voiding cystourethrography will demonstrate a wide-open proximal urethra in neurogenic conditions, and occlusion of the proximal urethra with obstruction at the time of a detrusor contraction.[26] Since prostatic enlargement appears to alter the sensorimotor balance of the central nervous system and to result in frequency, urgency, and nocturia, it is important to identify any obstructive component with involuntary detrusor contractions.

The Pathophysiology of Incontinence in the Elderly Male

As men become older, many changes occur in bladder function, including a decline in functional capacity.[8] Elderly incontinent patients have a lower functional bladder capacity than do similar continent patients.[8] As men become older, they usually describe getting up during the night to void. Approximately 70% of men over 65 years of age have symptoms of nocturia,[27] and it occurs much more frequently in those who are incontinent than in those who are not.[2, 28] This has important implications regarding the pathophysiology of incontinence. Nocturia occurs when the central sensory perception of a desire to void occurs while the individual is asleep and sleep arousal takes place without involuntary voiding. The observation of nocturia in incontinent patients appears inconsistent with the concept that these individuals lose the ability to inhibit the bladder. When nocturia occurs without involuntary urine loss, it suggests that central inhibition of the bladder is intact during sleep, sleep arousal, and voluntary voiding. If it were not, incontinence would occur. While the bladder may contract voluntarily during some episodes of nocturia, clearly incontinent patients lack the ability to inhibit the bladder every time. The inhibition of the bladder that occurs with nocturia has to be very strong in order to cause sleep arousal and avoid incontinence. During an event of nocturia in elderly incontinent patients, the bladder must remain inhibited while central nervous system awareness of a need to void occurs. This involuntary inhibition appears most likely to originate at a subcortical level; otherwise, incontinence would occur every time, since the individual is asleep and must be awakened by the event. Yet, incontinence does not occur regularly and voluntary nighttime voiding occurs frequently even in patients who have severe urinary incontinence. A patient's ability to retain bladder control at one time and not at another is important in understanding the pathophysiology of incontinence in the elderly.

Of all elderly patients who have urinary incontinence, 63% describe insufficient warning of the need to urinate, which seems to occur precipitously at any time.[28] Voluntary voiding episodes are associated with a sensation of a need to void that occurs well in advance of any bladder activity and allows the patient to void voluntarily. In elderly patients with urinary incontinence, voluntary and involuntary voiding are different events that occur at varying times in the same individual. With involuntary voiding, the perception of the impending or actual incontinence event is usually the first sensation that the patient has, while voluntary voiding is preceded by the perception of a need or desire to void. Therefore, there appears to be a difference in the sensory component of the voiding event from one episode to another. However, the complex events that occur neurologically during episodes of incontinence are unclear. Involuntary voiding may represent faulty perception of bladder sensation by the brain or the activation of a detrusor contraction from a site outside the normal bladder control centers of the brain. The difference in warning time before voiding described by the patient between incontinence and continence suggests that voluntary and involuntary events may occur in a different way and may be related in part to faulty brain perception of bladder fullness.

In our study of elderly men, incontinence measurements were performed in 66 inpatients over 10 days. An ambulatory electronic incontinence detection method allowed continuous nonobtrusive monitoring.[29-31] The inpatient environment allowed 24-hour monitoring of the frequency of incontinence episodes and the volume of involuntary urine loss. The highest total number of incontinence episodes occurred during the evening and the largest volume of involuntary urine loss occurred during the night.[30] The lowest frequency and volume of involuntary urine loss occurred during the day. The factors associated with this pattern were thought to be related to differences in fluid output and ambulation by the patient during the different times of the day.

From our study, a group of severely incontinent patients was selected for evaluation of the time interval between incontinence episodes. These continence intervals showed wide variations between episodes in all patients. Individual patients had incontinence episodes occurring less than 30 minutes apart as well as more than 6 hours apart. Thus, extremely irregular time intervals between episodes occurred within episodes for each patient. This irregularity within individuals suggests instability of the central nervous system sensorimotor regulatory mechanism of bladder control in all of the patients studied.[20] In addition to the variation in time intervals between episodes seen in severely incontinent patients, the volume per episode also was shown to be extremely variable.[32] Incontinence volumes of less than 25 mL to more than 350 mL were recorded in each case. This wide variability in volume per episode suggests that the occurrence of involuntary voiding in this group of elderly patients was independent of the intravesical volume at the time of the incontinence episode. Furthermore, the volume per episode of involuntary urine loss that occurred during routine daily activity of the patient was not related to the measured cystometric bladder capacity.

Because of the wide episodic variability in time between episodes and volume of urine loss per episode, a study of residual urine volume following involuntary voiding was performed.[33] The sum of the incontinence volume and the residual volume was considered to be equal to the total bladder volume at the time of an incontinence episode. Extreme variation was found in the incontinence volume, the residual urine volume, and the total bladder volume at the time of each incontinence episode. These data show that involuntary detrusor contractions in elderly incontinent men occur in an irregular manner and are independent of the accumulated volume of urine in the bladder.

Since the central nervous system responds to sensory information from the bladder, one possible explanation for the irregular activity of this organ in the elderly incontinent patient is failure of the central nervous system to integrate sensory information from the bladder and urethra properly in order to allow perception of the sensation of a need to void. Another possible explanation is that a stimulus for bladder contraction originates within the central nervous system, but outside the normal control pathways of bladder activity. In each of these cases, irregular bladder activity would occur without regard to the time interval since the last bladder contraction or the volume of urine accumulated within the bladder. In addition, little or no warning would be afforded the patient prior to the episode. Certainly, other explanations are possible, but additional insight awaits further studies on the neurophysiology of incontinence in this group of patients.

In preliminary studies using continuous telemetric monitoring of elderly incontinent men, we have recorded the external anal sphincter electromyogram (EMG), the intravesical pressure, the rectus abdominis EMG, and the occurrence of incontinence (Fig 1). Monitoring was done during the night in order to minimize the effect of changes in abdominal pressure on external anal sphincter EMG. In patients having stable central nervous system lesions resulting from a previous stroke, involuntary detrusor contractions have been observed during incontinence episodes as well as during episodic events in which incontinence was not detected. Abdominal pressure changes were not a factor in the increase in intravesical pressure shown since abdominal pressure changes show simultaneous changes in abdominal EMG, external sphincter EMG, and intravesical pressure as seen on the recording. The low amplitude of the external anal sphincter EMG associated with the detection of an incontinence event suggests that coordinated bladder-sphincter activity occurred during the incontinence episode. The involuntary detrusor contractions seen without incontinence

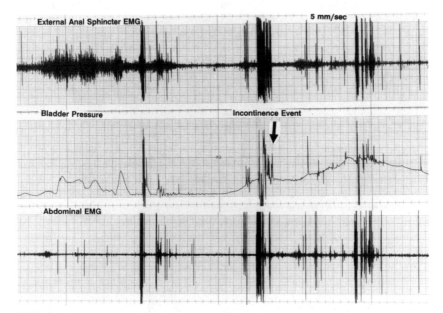

FIG 1.
Continuous telemetric monitoring of external anal sphincter EMG, intravesical pressure, rectus abdominis EMG, and incontinence detection is shown. Surface electrodes were used for EMG measurements, a 5-F infant feeding tube was placed through the urethra for monitoring of intravesical pressure, and electrical conductance across electrodes in a small absorbent pad at the urethral meatus was used to detect incontinence.

were associated with an increase in external sphincter EMG corresponding in amplitude to the changes in intravesical pressure. The detrusor contractions shown that are not associated with incontinence have a pattern consistent with detrusor-sphincter-dyssynergia. We have observed this pattern in patients who have no evidence of spinal cord disease. Additional studies need to be done to characterize these observations, but the preliminary observations suggest a possible CNS detrusor-sphincter reflex mechanism consisting of increased sphincteric activity and subsequent detrusor inhibition which can occur with episodes of involuntary detrusor contractions. Episodes of irregular detrusor-sphincter activity as described are consistent with the previous observations of irregular incontinence volume episodes and irregular incontinence intervals.

Another observation in elderly incontinent chronic care patients is the inability to void on command.[32, 33] This is seen frequently by nursing staff involved in incontinence treatment using a prompted voiding schedule for continence training. Elderly patients prompted to void and unable to do so often will experience urinary incontinence only minutes later, i.e., involuntary voiding frequently occurs when voluntary voiding could not be accomplished. Often, the intravesical volume at the time of the incontinence episode is adequate for voluntary voiding, but the patient's ability to do so appears to be impaired, making it difficult to measure a residual urine volume. The relationship of this deficit to incontinence is unclear. It seems that prompted voiding, which is the most common form of therapy used in elderly chronic care patients, may target the particular deficit of an inability to voluntarily initiate voiding. Pelvic floor exercise is another form of therapy commonly used in elderly incontinent patients. Contraction of the pelvic floor muscles reflexly inhibits the bladder. Pelvic floor exercises appear to target the particular deficit associated with urgency incontinence and detrusor instability.

Almost all elderly incontinent patients on some occasions void voluntarily, experience nocturia without incontinence, and describe normal sensations associated with voiding. These events indicate that the normal mechanisms of voiding and continence are functional in these patients, but are not always involved in the control of bladder activity.[34] In the elderly, there appears to exist an altered perception of the need to void or a lack of warning, an inability to inhibit or prevent involuntary voiding, and an inability to initiate voiding voluntarily.

In the elderly male who has not had previous prostate or pelvic surgery, stress urinary incontinence due to sphincteric incompetence is an unusual finding.[35] Sphincteric incompetence may occur following radical prostatectomy or an extensive abdominoperineal resection. In patients who have had abdominoperineal resection, all three of the elements of motor and sensory innervation of the genitourinary tract may be injured, including parasympathetic, sympathetic, and somatic innervation of the urethra.[36] These patients may void involuntarily in the upright position due to a loss of function of the urethral smooth muscle and skeletal sphincter resulting in stress incontinence due to sphincteric incompetence. Sphincteric incompetence also may be seen following radical prostatectomy. After radical prostatectomy, patients with urinary incontinence usually have stress incontinence with low maximum resting urethral pressure and negative pressure gradients with dynamic urethral pressure profilometry. Incontinence in these patients may be due in part to a partial denervation of the urethra that occurs during radical prostatectomy.[37] Postoperative changes in bladder compliance may be an additional factor in urinary incontinence following this procedure.[38] While sphincteric incompetence may occur following either radical prostatectomy or abdominoperineal resection, in the absence of previous pelvic surgery, sphincteric incompetence is rarely a factor in the etiology of incontinence in elderly men.

The Pathophysiology of Urinary Incontinence in the Elderly Female

As described previously, the incidence of urinary incontinence in community-dwelling elderly women is approximately 38%, about twice that of community-dwelling elderly men.[2, 16] Since women on an average have a much longer life span than do men in our society, the number of elderly women with incontinence is considerably greater than that of elderly men. For example, by the age of 85 years, there are only 40 men to every 100 women in the United States.[39] In chronic care facilities, females outnumber males by more than 2 to 1.[40] As women become older, cortical and physical impairment limit their activities and level of function in the same way as they do those of elderly men. Similarly, the functional disabilities of elderly women are also associated with a higher incidence of urinary incontinence. However, there is a major difference between the pathophysiology of incontinence in women and that in men. While sphincteric incompetence is an unusual cause of urinary incontinence in elderly men, it is the most common cause of incontinence in elderly women. In addition to sphincteric incompetence alone, the coexistence of sphincter incompetence, irritative bladder symptoms, and loss of central nervous system control of the bladder makes incontinence in many elderly females an extremely complex clinical problem.

In the early studies of elderly women by Brocklhurst,[6] 85% of the elderly incontinent women evaluated were found to have what he described as reflex or uninhibited neurogenic bladder contractions during filling cystometry. Numerous studies have been done since that time that have shown a similar high incidence of detrusor instability. In many cases, clinicians have made efforts to delineate further the difference between stress incontinence and urgency incontinence as an etiology of involuntary urine loss in these patients. However, after clinical evaluation of elderly women, some will have primarily stress incontinence due to sphincteric incompetence, some will have urgency incontinence associated with detrusor instability, and many will have components of both. The coexistence of irritative bladder symptoms and stress incontinence symptoms with urodynamic findings of both detrusor instability and sphincteric incompetence has become a well-recognized clinical entity. During patient evaluation, the described symptoms and urodynamic findings often suggest that the two problems may be related and possibly, a part of the same process.

In the past, it was believed that patients with stress incontinence generally should be approached surgically and that those with detrusor instability should be treated nonsurgically, since detrusor instability likely would continue to result in incontinence following surgery. However, that approach has changed considerably since McGuire described the disappearance in most cases of uninhibited detrusor dysfunction following incontinence surgery.[41-43] Many other urologists involved in surgery for female incontinence have confirmed this and since at the present time, the clinical identification of detrusor instability in association with stress urinary incontinence is of limited prognostic significance, it is likely to be ameliorated with surgery. Occasionally, some patients may experience irritative symptoms and detrusor instability only during the postoperative period.[42] Studies suggest that anatomic alterations in the urethra associated with stress incontinence also result in a disturbance of the sensorimotor balance of central nervous system control of the bladder in elderly female patients. The surgical correction of sphincteric incompetence in some way appears to stabilize this balance.

The Elderly Female Urethra

The two most important factors involved in competence of the female urethra are its anatomic support and the intrinsic closing properties of the urethral wall.[44] Changes in connective tissue surrounding the urethra occur with aging and can cause a loss of anatomic support of the proximal urethra and base of the bladder. In addition, the intrinsic urethral continence properties undergo marked changes as women become older. The spongy tissue of the submucosal layer of the urethra normally provides a mucosal seal in the proximal urethra that is necessary for continence. The abundant thin-walled venous sinuses and arterial venous connections in the submucosa contribute as much as 30% of urethral closure pressure.[45] This "vascular cushion" allows the efficient transmission of abdominal pressure changes to the urethra that are necessary for continence during episodes of increased abdominal pressure. The vascular component of the urethra is of such magnitude that urethral pressure profiles in young females often show pulsations at the peak of the profile that coincide with the arterial pulse. This appears to be due to arteriovenous shunting within the urethral wall.[46] These arterial pulsations of the urethra that are common in young women are not seen in elderly females. The reason for the decline in the vascular component of the urethra with aging is unclear, but is thought to be due in part to effects on the urethra of the changes in estrogen levels that occur with aging. An age relationship to maximum urethral closure pressure exists in women, with a steady decline as they become older.[47] Although the decline in maximum urethral closure pressure associated with aging is seen in both continent and incontinent women, it is considered to be a significant factor in the etiology of incontinence in the elderly.

In addition to estrogen deprivation, postmenopausal changes that affect the continence properties of the urethra may be due also to senescence or aging. Decreasing steroid production by the ovaries with advancing age results in senescent changes of the secondary sexual organs. The decline in production of these sex steroids, principally estradiol-17β, begins several years before menopause and is responsible for many changes that occur within the urethra apart from those resulting from the normal process of aging.

The lower urinary and reproductive tracts are of similar embryological origin.[48] Therefore, estrogens have a significant influence on the urethra, especially on the mucosa and submucosa. Estrogen receptors have been identified in the urethra, although they have not been demonstrated in the bladder. Lack of estrogen results in atrophic changes of the spongy tissue layer of the urethra in elderly women, with a loss of closing pressure and coaptation of the urethral mucosa that provides the seal necessary to maintain continence.[48]

Symptoms of stress incontinence and the urodynamic finding of sphincteric incompetence occur when the intraurethral pressure does not compensate adequately for increases in intra-abdominal pressure. When an elderly woman is standing or walking and has a sharp increase in intra-abdominal pressure due to coughing or straining, the intraurethral pressure responds with a sharp rise to maintain a closure pressure greater than the intra-abdominal and intravesical pressure. Because the cough transmission of pressure normally is more than 100% of the abdominal pressure, it has been concluded that there may be an active reflex phenomenon involved in the sharp intraurethral rise in pressure in response to the rise in abdominal pressure.[47] The proximal urethra is considered to be located normally within the abdominal cavity so that transmission of abdominal pressure to the proximal urethra allows a positive urethral closure pressure. Evidence exists for both a passive pressure transmission component within the proximal urethra and an active reflex pressure component. The compensatory functional pressure of the proximal urethra maintains an intraurethral pressure higher than the intravesical pressure at all times except during voiding. The dynamic change of the intraurethral pressure in response to changes in abdominal pressure is the central event that must be intact to prevent stress urinary incontinence. Alterations in the intrinsic properties of the urethra, such as atrophic changes in the submucosa and loss of anatomic support, interfere with the efficency of the normal compensatory pressure increases in the urethra and reduce its effectiveness. For example, dynamic urethral pressure profilometry in patients with stress incontinence shows that a positive pressure response to increased intra-abdominal pressure actually occurs in almost all patients. The intraurethral pressure increase in response to increased intra-abdominal pressure in these patients shows that the compensatory pressure mechanism of the urethra is active, but the magnitude of the response is inadequate to maintain a positive pressure gradient between the urethra and bladder. The single urethral pressure parameter that shows significant change following surgery for stress incontinence is the restoration of the positive pressure gradient in the proximal urethra.[49] The compensatory rise in urethral pressure in response to changes in intra-abdominal pressure that was present prior to surgery, but inadequate to maintain a positive pressure gradient, becomes more efficient following surgery and a positive pressure gradient results. The objective of female stress incontinence procedures appears to be alteration of the intrinsic and extrinsic anatomic configuration of the urethra in such a way that the pressure compensating activity of the urethra is more efficient and a positive pressure gradient between the proximal urethra and bladder is maintained at all times.

The many intrinsic and extrinsic changes that occur following incontinence surgery that produce continence are not completely understood. Investigative anatomic studies of the urethra using magnetic resonance imaging currently are being done and have provided a better understanding of the anatomic abnormalities of the urethra associated with incontinence and the changes that occur following surgery. The outcome of these studies will be valuable in the future for further elucidation of the anatomic changes in the lower urinary tract that are associated with incontinence and aging.[50]

Summary

The medical, social, economic, and psychological impact of urinary incontinence on the elderly is immense, for both individuals in the community and those in chronic care facilities. The effects of aging alter the anatomy and physiology of the lower urinary tract in many ways that can contribute significantly to a loss of continence. Central nervous system control of the bladder appears to play a major role in the pathophysiology of incontinence in the elderly and much research effort will be required to understand better the mechanisms that are involved. There are many similarities between incontinence in elderly men and elderly women. However, stress incontinence associated with sphincteric incompetence and urgency symptoms with detrusor instability in the elderly female makes treatment an especially difficult and complex problem to manage. With the advancing age of our society, the problem of urinary incontinence will require the development of appropriate therapeutic options by clinicians and researchers.

References

1. *Urinary Incontinence in Adults: National Institutes of Health Consensus Development Conference Statement,* vol 7, 1988 pp 1–27.
2. Diokno AC, Brock BM, Brown MB, et al: Prevalence of urinary incontinence and other urological symptoms in the noninstitutionalized elderly. *J Urol* 1986; 136:1022–1025.

3. Ehrman JS: Correspondence from Washington, use of biofeedback to treat incontinence. *J Am Geriatr Soc* 1983; 31:182–184.
4. Resnick NM, Yalla SV, Laurino E: Urinary incontinence among elderly persons. *New Engl J Med* 1989; 320:1421–1422.
5. Wilson TS: Incontinence of urine in the aged. *Lancet* 1948; 255:374–377.
6. Brocklhurst JC, Dillane JB: Studies of the female bladder in old age II. Cystometrograms in 100 incontinent women. *Gerontol Clin* 1966; 8:306–319.
7. Isaacs B, Walkey FA: A survey of incontinence in elderly hospital patients. *Gerontol Clin* 1964; 6:367–376.
8. Brocklhurst JC: The management of incontinence. *Postgrad Med J* 1967; 43:527–533.
9. Kock NG, Pompeius R: Inhibition of vesical motor activity induced by anal stimulation. *Acta Chir Sand* 1963; 126:244–250.
10. O'Shaughnessy EJ, Clowers DE, Brooks G: Detrusor reflex contraction inhibited by anal stretch. *Arch Phys Med Rehabil* 1981; 62:128–130.
11. Ouslander J: Incontinence. *Maryland Medical Journal* 1989; 38:130–132.
12. Walkey FA, Judge TG, Thompson J, et al: Incidence of urinary infection in the elderly. *Scot Med J* 1967; 12:411–414.
13. Bosica JA, Kobasa WD, Abrutyn E, et al: Lack of association between bacteriuria and symptoms in the elderly. *Am J Med* 1986; 81:979–982.
14. Ouslander JG, Uman GC, Urman HN, et al: Incontinence among nursing home patients: Clinical and functional correlates. *J Am Geriatr Soc* 1987; 35:324–330.
15. Ouslander JG, Kane RL, Abrass IB: Urinary incontinence in elderly nursing home patients. *JAMA* 1982; 248:1194–1198.
16. Teasdale TA, Taffett GE, Luchi RJ, et al: Urinary incontinence in a community-residing elderly population. *J Am Geriatr Soc* 1988; 36:600–606.
17. Campbell AJ, Reinken J, McCosh L: Incontinence in the elderly: Prevalence and prognosis. *Age Ageing* 1985; 14:65–70.
18. Wade DT, Hewer RL: Outlook after an acute stroke: Urinary incontinence and loss of consciousness compared in 532 patients. *J Med* 1985; 56:601–608.
19. Robb SS: Urinary incontinence verification in elderly men. *Nurs Res* 1985; 34:278–282.
20. O'Donnell PD: Continence interval in elderly incontinent men. *Neurourology and Urodynamics* 1989; 8:505–511.
21. Castleden CM, Duffin HM, Asher MJ: Clinical and urodynamic studies in 100 elderly incontinent patients. *Br Med J* 1981; 282:1103–1105.
22. Overstall PW, Rounce K, Palmer JH: Experience with an incontinence clinic. *J Am Geriatr Soc* 1980; 28:535–538.
23. Ouslander JG, Hepps K, Raz S, et al: Genitourinary dysfunction in a geriatric outpatient population. *J Am Geriatr Soc* 1986; 34:507–513.
24. McGrother CW, Castleden CM, Duffin H, et al: A profile of disordered micturition in the elderly at home. *Age Ageing* 1987; 16:105–110.
25. Diokno AC, Morton BB, Brock BM, et al: Clinical and cystometric characteristics of continent and incontinent noninstitutionalized elderly. *J Urol* 1988; 140:567–571.
26. McGuire EJ: Urinary dysfunction in the aged: Neurological considerations. *Bull N Y Acad Med* 1980; 56:275–284.
27. Brocklehurst JC, Fry J, Griffiths LL, et al: Dysuria in old age. *J Am Geriatr Soc* 1971; 19:582–592.
28. Barker JC, Mitteness LS: Nocturia in the elderly. *J Gerontological Soc Am* 1988; 28:99–104.

29. O'Donnell PD, Marshall MF: Telemetric ambulatory urinary incontinence detection in the elderly. *J Ambulatory Monitoring* 1988; 1:233–240.
30. O'Donnell PD, Beck C, Walls RC: Serial incontinence assessment in elderly inpatient men. *J Rehabil Res Dev* 1990; 27:1–8.
31. O'Donnell PD, Sutton LE, Beck CM, et al: Urinary incontinence detection in elderly inpatient men. *Neurourology and Urodynamics* 1987; 6:101–108.
32. O'Donnell PD, Beck C: Urinary incontinence volume patterns in elderly inpatient men. *Urology,* in press.
33. Starer P, Libow LS: The measurement of residual urine in the evaluation of incontinent nursing home residents. *Arch Gerontol Geriatr* 1988; 7:75–81.
34. O'Donnell PD, Walls RC: Residual urine volume following involuntary voiding in elderly inpatient men. *Neurourology and Urodynamics* 1990; 9:35–42.
35. Woodside JR: Stress urinary incontinence in men. *J Urol* 1982; 128:1246–1249.
36. McGuire EJ: Neurovesical dysfunction after abdominoperineal resection. *Surg Clin North Am* 1980; 60:1207–1213.
37. O'Donnell PD, Finan BF: Continence following nerve sparing radical prostatectomy. *J Urol* 1989; 142:1227–1229.
38. Leach GE, Yip CM, Donovan BJ: Mechanism of continence after modified pereyra bladder neck suspension. *Urology* 1987; 29:148–179.
39. *Aging America: Trends and Projections.* Rockville, Md, US Department of Health and Human Services, Publication No LR 3377 188 D 12198, 1987–1988.
40. Wells TJ, Brink CA, Diokno AC: Urinary incontinence in elderly women: Clinical findings. *J Am Geriatr Soc* 1987; 35:933–939.
41. McGuire EJ, Lytton B: Pubovaginal sling procedure for stress incontinence. *J Urol* 1978; 119:82–84.
42. McGuire EJ, Lytton B, Kohorn EI, et al: The value of urodynamic testing in stress urinary incontinence. *J Urol* 1980; 124:256–258.
43. McGuire EJ: Urinary incontinence in the elderly. *J Arkansas Med Soc* 1985; 81:640–642.
44. Schmidbauer CP, Chiang H, Raz S: Surgical treatment for female geriatric incontinence. *Clin Geriatr Med* 1986; 2:759–776.
45. Staskin DR, Zimmern PE, Hadley HR, et al: The pathophysiology of stress incontinence. *Urol Clin North Am* 1985; 12:271–278.
46. Bruskewitz RR: Urethral pressure profile in female lower urinary tract dysfunction, in Raz (ed): *Female Urology.* Philadelphia, WB Saunders, 1983, pp 113–122.
47. Constantinou CE: Resting and stress urethral pressures as a clinical guide to the mechanism of continence in the female patient. *Urol Clin North Am* 1985; 12:247–258.
48. Corlett RC: Age-specific urinary tract problems, in Buschbaum, Schmidt (eds): *Gynecologic and Obstetric Urology.* Philadelphia, WB Saunders, 1982, pp 387–394.
49. Leach GE, Yip CM: Urologic and urodynamic evaluation of the elderly population. *Clin Geriatr Med* 1986; 2:731–755.
50. Klutke C, Golomb J, Barbaric Z, et al: The anatomy of stress incontinence: Magnetic resonance imaging of the female bladder neck and urethra. *J Urol* 1990; 143:563–566.

The Diagnosis of Renal Hypertension

Mark C. Saddler, M.B.Ch.B.

Westchester County Foundation, Fellow in Hypertension, Yale University School of Medicine, New Haven, Connecticut

Henry R. Black, M.D.

Professor of Internal Medicine, Director, Preventive Cardiology Service, Yale University School of Medicine, New Haven, Connecticut

Hypertension is the most frequent reason that Americans see their physicians; almost 60 million of us have an elevated blood pressure.[1] It is a major risk factor for premature mortality, coronary artery disease, congestive heart failure, cerebrovascular disease, and peripheral vascular disease. Hypertension usually is considered to be either essential (primary), for which a cause is unknown, or secondary, for which a cause can be identified. Although the overwhelming majority of the hypertensive population has essential hypertension, there is still a sizable subgroup of patients who have a secondary cause for an elevated blood pressure (Table 1). The actual percentage of hypertensives with a secondary cause is difficult to determine, with estimates ranging between 0.5% and 10%.[2-5]

Excluding drug-induced (iatrogenic) hypertension, diseases of the kidney are the most common causes of secondary hypertension. Renal parenchymal disease is a more common cause of hypertension than are diseases of the renal vasculature, but the latter is very important for three reasons. First, it may be difficult to control the blood pressure successfully with medications in a patient with renovascular hypertension (RVH). Second, in contrast to renal parenchymal disease, RVH is often curable. Although many patients still require surgery (either a revascularization or a nephrectomy), the advent of renal angioplasty has allowed those who previously had been unable or unwilling to withstand the stress of an operation to be treated successfully.[6, 7] Finally, renal ischemia due to renal artery obstructive lesions frequently progresses to chronic renal failure.

A significant number of patients who develop end-stage renal disease as a result of arterial obstruction may be able to avoid or delay chronic dialysis or renal transplantation if a renal revascularization procedure is performed while the kidney is still viable. In a recent series of Schreiber et al., progression of atherosclerotic renal artery stenosis (RAS) occurred in 44% of patients with this lesion, and the serum creatinine increased by more than 20% in 38% of the cases.[8] Other authors have reported a similar fre-

TABLE 1.
Causes of Secondary
Hypertension

I. Renal disease.
  A. Parenchymal (chronic renal failure).
  B. Vascular (RAS).
II. Endocrine disease.
  A. Primary aldosteronism.
  B. Pheochromocytoma.
  C. Hyperthyroidism.
  D. Hyperparathyroidism.
  E. Cushing's syndrome.
III. Coarctation of the aorta.
IV. Iatrogenic.
  A. Nonsteroidal anti-inflammatory
     agents.
  B. Oral contraceptives.
  C. Sympathomimetic amines.
  D. Cyclosporine.
  E. Erythropoietin.
V. Pregnancy.

quency of progression.[9, 10] If renal perfusion is restored by adequate revascularization in these patients, the inexorable progression to end-stage renal disease may be delayed or even prevented.

Though this discussion will focus on hypertension due to diseases of the renal vasculature, rather than that associated with renal parenchymal disease, it should be noted that the two diseases may occur in the same patient. Patients with renal parenchymal disease may develop RVH, but more frequently, patients with RVH develop renal insufficiency due to renal ischemia and may come to medical attention because of an elevated creatinine rather than because of hypertension.

Before discussing our approach to evaluating patients suspected of having RVH, it is important to emphasize that the presence of an anatomic lesion in the renal artery does not necessarily mean that hypertension in that patient is the result of that lesion. RAS simply means an anatomic narrowing of the renal artery (due to atheromatous plaque, fibromuscular disease, or other causes). The patient with RAS need not have hypertension, or if he or she does, it may not be due to RAS. In one study, as many as 49% of elderly *normotensive* individuals had RAS.[11] The term "renovascular hypertension," on the other hand, specifies that the hypertension is present *as a result of RAS*. The only way to be certain that this is the case is to restore or improve perfusion by surgery or angioplasty and demonstrate improvement or cure. The Cooperative Study of Renovascular Hypertension, the largest study of this disorder to date, carefully defined patients as having "proved," "probable," or "possible" RVH[12] (Table 2). Therefore, the renal arteriogram, though currently our best means of visualizing the anatomy of the renal arteries, has the significant disadvantage of telling us little about the functional significance of any lesion observed.

Our basic approach to the diagnosis of RVH is as follows. First, we limit evaluation to only those patients to whom we would offer revascularization or angioplasty should a lesion be found. Second, we recognize that most hypertensive patients do not have RVH and that any noninvasive diagnostic test we choose will have a low predictive value if applied to the unselected population of all hypertensives. Therefore, we select patients for investigation for RVH based on clinical factors. Last, we still conclude our diagnostic work-up with arteriography in any patient in whom our index of

---

TABLE 2.
Definition and Classification of Renovascular Hypertension According to the Cooperative Study of Renovascular Hypertension

I. Patients initially evaluated.
  A. Proved.
    1. Patients who respond favorably to operative treatment, i.e., are cured or improved.
  B. Probable.
    1. Patients with many of the diagnostic parameters of curable (proved) renovascular hypertension whose failure to respond to surgery can be explained by other factors or who have not undergone corrective surgery.
  C. Possible.
    1. Patients with many of the diagnostic parameters of curable (proved) renovascular hypertension whose failure to respond to surgery is unexplained.
II. Patients surviving surgery and evaluated 12 months or more postoperatively.
  A. Cured.
    1. Patients with average diastolic blood pressure of 90 mm Hg or less and with at least 10 mm Hg decrease from the preoperative level.
  B. Improved.
    1. Patients with a 15% or greater decrease in average diastolic blood pressure, and whose diastolic blood pressure is greater than 90 mm Hg but less than 110 mm Hg.
  C. Failure.
    1. Patients with less than a 15% decrease in average diastolic blood pressure, and whose diastolic blood pressure is greater than 90 mm Hg.
    2. Patients with a diastolic blood pressure greater than 110 mm Hg.

suspicion that the disease is present is high. No test currently available is specific enough to exclude RVH with 100% certainty. As we will discuss, the discovery of a renal artery lesion is only the beginning of our diagnostic dilemma. The real problem is to try to distinguish those renal artery lesions that are responsible for the patient's hypertension from those that are not.

Clinical Features

None of the diagnostic tests we have for RVH replace a careful history and physical examination. Clinical clues can be of great value in helping to select high-risk patients from the general hypertensive population. The clinical features that should raise suspicion of RVH are listed in Table 3. One of the most important features of the history is to ascertain the presence of previous or current vascular disease in other arterial beds. Similarly, physical examination for vascular disease is vital and should include careful auscultation of the carotid and femoral arteries for bruits. Should an abdominal bruit be present, it is a very valuable sign suggestive of RVH. However, the majority of patients with RAS do not have this finding.[13]

TABLE 3.
Typical Clinical Features of Renal Artery Stenosis (RAS)

I. Fibromuscular dysplasia.
   A. Age <35 years.
   B. Caucasian.
   C. Female gender.
   D. Cigarette smoking.
   E. Abdominal bruits.
   F. Resistant or severe hypertension.
   G. Renal dysfunction.
II. Atherosclerotic RAS.
   A. Age >55 years.
   B. Caucasian.
   C. Male gender.
   D. Vascular disease in coronary, cerebral, or peripheral arteries.
   E. Cigarette smoking.
   F. Abdominal bruits.
   G. Resistant or severe hypertension.
   H. Renal dysfunction.

Biochemical Tests

A number of simple biochemical parameters help in determining which patients need more extensive investigation. An elevated creatinine is common with bilateral RAS. Hypokalemia, especially that unassociated with diuretic therapy, occurs more commonly in patients with RVH than in those with essential hypertension, due to increased activity of the renin-angiotensin-aldosterone system. This "secondary aldosteronism" increases potassium secretion by the kidney. Simon et al. found that a serum potassium level below 3.4 mEq/L occurred in less than 20% of cases.[14] This association was not found in Anderson's series.[15] Similarly, hyperuricemia[16] and elevation of the hematocrit[17] have been proposed as markers of the disease, but are of limited value in practice.

Renin

The value of measuring plasma renin activity (PRA) remains a complex and controversial issue. Renin is secreted by the macula densa in response to decreased delivery of chloride to the distal tubule.[18] This situation occurs in the presence of a hemodynamically significant stenosis of a renal artery. Renin secretion increases the secretion of angiotensin and aldosterone, raising the blood pressure. However, even the most precise methods of measuring PRA have failed to allow this test to realize its theoretical promise for diagnosing RVH. This may be because renin achieves its effect through local action within the kidney and this is not always reflected by the level of renin in the plasma. In addition, the renin assay technique is difficult to perform and affected by posture, volume status, and drugs. Only centers that perform the test frequently show reproducible results. Normal laboratory processing can cause conversion of the inactive circulating prorenin into active renin, further confounding the significance of the measured PRA.[19]

Furthermore, it increasingly is being realized that the action of angiotensin is not necessarily dependent on renin. Other proteases, such as the cathepsins, appear capable of converting angiotensinogen to angiotensin I and even angiotensin II directly.[20] This puts the physiological role of renin in further question and explains why its measurement has been a disappointing indicator of RVH.

Peripheral Blood Plasma Renin Activity

Rudnick and Maxwell's review of 24 published series of measurements of peripheral blood PRA is illuminating and demonstrates some of the problems associated with this technique.[21] Although 86% of patients with an elevated PRA were improved by surgery, so were 71% of patients with a normal PRA. The overall sensitivity of the test was 57% and the specificity was 66%.

Because of these problems, recently there has been much interest in the technique of renin *stimulation* by angiotensin-converting enzyme (ACE) inhibitors. Laragh's group at Cornell University[22] used the following criteria for a positive test result:

1. Stimulated PRA (60 minutes after captopril 50 mg orally) of 12 ng/mL/hr or more *and,*
2. Absolute increase in PRA of 10 ng/mL/hr or more *and,*
3. 150% or greater increase in PRA following captopril (400% or greater increase if baseline PRA <3 ng/mL/hr).

Using these criteria, they claimed 100% sensitivity and 95% specificity for the test. However, the study suffered from the following limitations:

1. Not all of the patients in the control group underwent arteriography. Therefore, RVH was not definitely excluded in these patients.
2. The stated figures for sensitivity and specificity pertained only to patients with normal renal function. In patients with renal impairment, the accuracy of the test was much lower; 31% of their patients labeled as nonrenovascular hypertensives had a positive result in this group.
3. The data were collected on a retrospective basis.
4. Antihypertensive medications were discontinued for 3 weeks prior to the test, subjecting patients to considerable risk.

Two subsequent European studies have found stimulated peripheral PRA to be a poor diagnostic test. Salvetti et al. found the sensitivity of the test to be only 20%,[23] while Idrissi et al., following similarly poor results, suggested that the main use of the test might be to help establish the significance of a lesion already shown by arteriography.[24] In contrast, Derkx et al.[25] found that the test had a sensitivity of 93% and a specificity of 84%. Their technique was similar to that used by Idrissi and Salvetti and it is not clear why these differences in results were obtained. More recently, two more studies have come to different conclusions regarding the value of stimulated peripheral PRA. Postma et al. studied 149 patients, found a sensitivity of 39%, and concluded that the test was unsuitable for screening.[26] In contrast, Frederickson et al. achieved a sensitivity of 100% and a specificity of 80%.[27] However, not all of Frederickson's patients labeled "non-RVH" or essential hypertensives had arteriograms (in fact, only 21% of them did). Therefore, the real sensitivity of the method in his team's hands cannot be definitely determined. In the absence of good data demonstrating the value of this test, we currently do not recommend it in the routine investigation of patients with suspected RVH.

At the same time as measuring stimulated peripheral PRA, a number of workers have looked at changes in blood pressure following a single dose of captopril. In theory, patients with RVH should be maximally angiotensin-dependent for maintenance of their elevated blood pressure. An ACE inhibitor, therefore, would be expected to have a more profound effect in lowering the blood pressure of a patient with RVH than that of a patient with essential hypertension. Although Marks et al. described some cases in whom this technique was useful,[28] most investigators have found the procedure to be of limited accuracy.[22]

Renal Vein Renin

Numerous investigators have turned to sampling PRA from the renal veins to improve the predictive accuracy of renin levels. This procedure has been evaluated as a predictor of significant renal artery occlusion and to determine which patients have a lesion curable by surgery or angioplasty. It has been suggested that the elevated PRA found in the renal vein of a stenotic kidney is a consequence of both increased secretion and decreased flow.[29] Most clinicians use a ratio of PRA between the two renal veins of 1.5 or greater to indicate a "positive" test result with a high likelihood of RAS. However, the 95% confidence limit for renal vein renin ratios in essential hypertensive populations is probably closer to 2.0,[30] and this figure has been suggested as a more appropriate ratio to reduce false-positive results.[31] Unfortunately, a significant number of patients with both essential hypertension and RVH have renal vein renin ratios between 1.0 and 2.0, reducing the usefulness of the test. Evaluating bilateral disease can be difficult with this technique; eliciting a positive test result depends on a degree of asymmetry of secretion, since even severe bilateral disease would not produce a lateralizing ratio if both sides secreted high, but equal, amounts of renin. Secretion of renin varies from minute to minute, so it has been suggested that each renal vein be catheterized and renin sampled simultaneously from each side.[32]

Vaughan et al.[33] devised a scoring system to improve the reliability of the test, using three criteria: (1) abnormally high peripheral PRA in relation to sodium excretion, (2) complete suppression of renin from one kidney, and (3) increased renal vein PRA compared with arterial PRA from the other kidney. This method improved the accuracy, but increased the complexity of interpreting the results and necessitated an arterial puncture.

Again, Rudnick and Maxwell's review of 58 published series investigating renal vein PRA is helpful.[21] Most of these series considered a ratio of 1.5 or greater to be a positive result. Analyzing all of the trials together showed that a positive test result correctly predicted improvement following surgery in 92% of cases, even when bilateral disease was present. However, 65% of cases with a nonlateralizing renal vein renin also achieved improvement following surgery. This constitutes an unacceptably high false-negative predictive value and renders a negative test result virtually uninterpretable.[30, 34]

Similar to the situation with peripheral PRA, several methods have been tried to improve the predictive value of renal vein renin ratios by stimulating renin release. Various techniques used have included changes of posture,[35] salt depletion,[36] and the infusion of vasodilators including hydralazine[37] and diazoxide.[38] Recently, the ACE inhibitors have been used by several groups for this purpose.

In 1978, Re et al. reported that ACE inhibitors increased the PRA concentration in the vein of the ischemic kidney while slightly reducing the renal venous PRA concentration from the contralateral nonstenotic kidney.[39] This might be expected, since the underperfused ischemic kidney requires angiotensin II to maintain its glomerular filtration rate. If the effect of the angiotensin II is withdrawn using an ACE inhibitor, the glomerular filtration rate would be expected to drop in that kidney, with a resultant increase in renin production. Re's results were confirmed later by Thibonnier et al.[40] Lyons subsequently showed that the use of captopril to stimulate the secretion of renin in patients with RAS improved the accuracy of renal vein renin ratios.[41] He looked at 26 patients and compared their renal vein renin ratio at baseline with their ratio 30 minutes after a 25-mg oral dose of captopril. A stimulated renal vein renin ratio of 3.0 or greater was considered positive. Similar results were found in a smaller series from Israel.[42] Morganti et al. in addition looked at the secretion of both active and inactive forms of renin following captopril administration.[43] Not only was the secretion of total renin from the stenotic kidney increased, but the ratio of active to inactive renin also increased.

The use of stimulated renal vein renin ratios, therefore, shows some promise in the diagnosis of RVH. However, two important disadvantages are associated with this test. First, it necessitates the manipulation of a catheter into the renal veins and second, the accuracy of the results depends on the skill of the institution performing the PRA measurements in the blood samples submitted.

Split Renal Function Studies

Bilateral ureteral catheterization has been used to diagnose RVH in the past. The ureters are selectively catheterized at cystoscopy; the urine flow and composition from each kidney then can be measured independently. Criteria that have been used to indicate a positive test result include a 3:1 ratio of urine flow rates,[44] 100% or greater difference in concentration of para-amino hippuric acid,[44] 50% higher creatinine concentration from the affected side,[45] or a 15% reduction in sodium concentration on the affected side.[45] Trials of this technique generally have been favorable, especially with respect to the prediction of surgical cure.[46] However, it has fallen from use to a large extent because of the invasiveness of the procedure. Some of the information previously obtained by this technique now can be elicited by radionuclide methods of split renal function testing.

Renal Biopsy

Biopsy of the affected kidney, and sometimes even both kidneys, has been tried as a method of predicting the presence of RAS. The major problems with this method are the trauma and risks involved and the lack of specific histological findings associated with RAS. Hyperplasia of the juxtaglomerular apparatus has been suggested as a distinguishing criterion,[47, 48] but even this finding is not sensitive or specific enough to justify performing a renal biopsy to make the diagnosis of curable RVH.

Imaging Methods

Important advances in the diagnosis of RVH have been made through imaging methods in recent years. The renal arteriogram remains the "gold standard" against which all other tests currently are measured. Any patient for whom an interventional procedure is planned will require an arteriogram to delineate the position and extent of a stenotic lesion. Even if any of the other tests were perfectly accurate in predicting which patients have RVH, an arteriogram would still be necessary in patients who tested positive before proceeding to operation or angioplasty. No other test (with the exception of ultrasonography) visualizes the anatomic characteristics of a stenotic lesion. The role of imaging procedures other than arteriography, therefore, should be to identify those patients who *do not* have the disease. It is hoped that, in this way, a number of patients will be spared the discomfort, expense, and risk of renal arteriography.

Contrast nephropathy and cholesterol embolization are the major risks to the kidney of renal arteriography. The likelihood of the former appears to be reduced substantially if the dose of contrast is kept as low as possible.[49] Hopes that the newer nonionic contrast agents would prove less nephrotoxic are not supported by hard experimental evidence.[50, 51] Renal dysfunction due to contrast agents unfortunately is more common in diabetic patients and those with renal dysfunction—two groups in whom one would expect RVH to be more common.[52] When considering such patients for arteriography, the risks must be weighed carefully against the potential benefits. One possible method of reducing the risk of contrast nephropathy might be the use of calcium channel blockers prior to administration of the contrast agent.[53] Initial studies of the value of these agents in this situation appear promising. Adequate hydration prior to the procedure also seems a sensible precaution.

Intravenous digital subtraction angiography evolved as a less invasive means of making the diagnosis of RAS. Despite some promise,[54, 56] good visualization of the renal arteries is not achieved in some patients and this contributes to a high false-positive rate (26% to 37% in one series).[56] The risk of contrast nephropathy remains present with this procedure and patients with positive results often require an arteriogram anyway before correction of the stenosis can be performed. For these reasons, we have abandoned this procedure at our institution. However, whenever possible, we use the technique of intra-arterial digital subtraction angiography as a useful way of limiting the dose of contrast material required to visualize the renal arteries.

Although renal arteriography gives information regarding the anatomy of a stenosis that no other test currently can match, it provides little information about the hemodynamic significance of the lesions it demonstrates. It seems intuitively reasonable that the greater the degree of anatomic stenosis, the more likely the lesion is to be hemodynamically significant. For research purposes, we arbitrarily have considered 75% or greater stenoses to be hemodynamically significant. In addition, a 50% or greater stenosis has been considered significant in our trial if accompanied by poststenotic dilation. Some of the tests described as follows, which depend on various functional changes within the kidney, may provide more useful information in this regard.

Intravenous Pyelography

The intravenous pyelogram (IVP) was first used for the purpose of identifying patients with RVH in the early 1960s,[57, 58] but is now sliding into obsolescence as the nuclear scanning techniques improve. During a "rapid sequence" or "hypertensive" urogram, radiographs of the kidney are taken at 1, 2, 3, 4, and 30 minutes. The changes seen on the IVP that indicate an increased likelihood of RVH are shown in Table 4.[59] These changes are the markers of two pathophysiological processes resulting from RAS: decreased blood flow and the concentration of urine.

The Radiology Study Group of the Cooperative Study of Renovascular Hypertension concluded in 1972, and subsequently in 1977, that urography was a "satisfactory" screening test.[60, 61] However, subsequent studies have not shown such favorable results. Thornbury et al. found that only 24% of patients with a positive urogram had a favorable surgical outcome and that the false-negative rate was as high as 22%.[62] In addition to these disadvantages relating to poor accuracy, patients undergoing urography are exposed to contrast, with its attendant risk of nephrotoxicity.

TABLE 4.
Intravenous Pyelogram Findings Suggestive of Renovascular Hypertension

Difference in renal lengths >1.5
Delayed urogram
Delayed onset, prolonged duration, and
    hyperconcentration of nephrogram
Ureteral notching
Decreased size of pyelocalyceal system
    ("spidery" calyces)
Delayed "washout" during diuresis

Ultrasound and Doppler

A renal ultrasound examination can be a useful test in a patient with suspected RVH. Differences in renal size frequently will indicate a need for further investigation. Indeed, a difference in renal size, demonstrated by an ultrasound examination performed for a different reason, frequently leads to the first suspicion of RAS in a patient. The test is neither sensitive nor specific enough to be used for a screening, but whenever one small kidney is seen on ultrasound, the clinician should always consider RAS in the differential diagnosis.

Duplex Doppler and color Doppler ultrasound imaging have been applied to the renal arteries in an attempt to visualize stenoses. Areas of stenosis show an increase in blood velocity and turbulence. The region of maximum disturbance to flow may be localized using color Doppler imaging.[63] Though many different criteria for the diagnosis of RAS using Doppler techniques have been proposed (Table 5), the most reliable method

TABLE 5.
Results of Previous Studies Investigating the Use of Duplex Doppler Ultrasound to Identify Patients With Renovascular Hypertension

Author	Reference	Year	Number	Criteria for Positive Examination	Results
Avasthi	64	1984	26	Peak blood velocity >100 cm/sec Absence of diastolic flow Absence of any flow (occlusion) Broad-band Doppler frequency spectra	Sensitivity 89% Specificity 73%
Norris	65	1984	120*	Elevated systolic frequency Spectral broadening	Sensitivity 83% Specificity 97%
Kohler	66	1986	22	Ratio of peak velocities in renal artery vs. aorta >3.5	Sensitivity 91%
Taylor	67	1987	29	Ratio of peak velocity in renal artery vs. aorta >3.5	Sensitivity 84% Specificity 97%
Strandness	68	1990	58	Ratio of peak velocity in renal artery vs. aorta >3.5	Specificity 97%

*Attempted in 120 patients; successful in 112 patients.

relies on the ratio of the peak systolic velocity in the renal artery to the peak systolic in the aorta. If this ratio is greater than 3.5, there is a high likelihood that RAS is present.

Doppler ultrasound techniques have potential advantages as tools for predicting RAS. The procedure is devoid of risk or significant discomfort to the patient. Moreover, because it involves observing characteristics of flow, it theoretically might provide information about the hemodynamic significance of a lesion, rather than merely about the anatomic configuration of an arterial narrowing. However, there are some drawbacks. First, the procedure is very operator-dependent, requiring a skilled ultrasonographer who has had significant experience with the technique.[69] Second, the renal vasculature cannot be imaged in every patient in whom the diagnosis of RAS is considered; one recent report found that 40% of examinations were inadequate.[63] The most common reasons for failure to visualize the renal arteries were obesity, excessive bowel gas, recent surgical procedure, aortic aneurysm, and eating prior to the examination. Third, even when the Doppler ultrasound examination is successful, there are some technical limitations; the distal portion of the artery is difficult to visualize, as are accessory renal arteries. Collateral vessels also have caused confusion in interpretation.[66] However, the technique may be more useful in identifying RVH in transplanted kidneys, since the allograft's circulation is more accessible to ultrasonic examination.[70]

Scintigraphic Methods

Since radionuclide scintigraphy provides reliable measurements of each separate kidney's function in a noninvasive manner, it would seem the logical way to investigate patients for the presence of RAS. However, initial results using ^{131}I-iodohippurate were disappointing. In 1975, the report of the Cooperative Study of Renovascular Hypertension revealed unacceptable 25% false-positive and 24% false-negative rates.[71] Subsequent studies using different isotopes proved somewhat more successful, and Chiarini et al. found that the use of ^{99m}Tc-diethylenetriaminepentaacetic acid (DTPA) gave a sensitivity of 90% and a specificity of 91% in his group of patients.[72] Similarly, Gross et al. found that DTPA was more useful than ^{131}I-iodohippurate in identifying patients with RAS.[73] Another group found that ^{99m}Tc-glucoheptonate was also a useful radioisotope in the initial diagnosis and follow-up of patients with RAS.[74] However, such baseline renal scanning can demonstrate only a decrease in glomerular filtration rate or effective renal plasma flow. The cause of these alterations in function cannot be deduced from the results of the scan alone. Therefore, a kidney malfunctioning from any cause (e.g., prolonged obstruction, pyelonephritis, congenital dysplasia, etc.) cannot be distinguished from a kidney with RAS. This would be expected to contribute to the number of false-positive results. Moreover, even a kidney with significant RAS may be able to compensate sufficiently through activation of the renin-angiotensin system so that alterations in its function cannot be identified by scintigraphy. This shortcoming presumably adds to the false-negative rate. Therefore, a number of groups recently have investigated the use of ACE inhibitors prior to scintigraphy in an attempt to solve these problems.

Angiotensin is a potent vasoconstrictor.[75] In the kidney it causes greater constriction of the efferent than the afferent glomerular arteriole, thus maintaining the glomerular filtration rate.[76] In a patient with RAS, the decreased renal perfusion would cause a fall in this rate were it not for the action of angiotensin. Such a kidney would be expected to experience a profound decrease in the glomerular filtration rate following the administration of an ACE inhibitor. Therefore, by performing first a baseline renal scintigram and then another scan after administering an ACE inhibitor, one would expect to see a fall in the rate in a kidney with hemodynamically significant RAS on the second scan.[77] This is the rationale underlying what has come to be known as the "captopril scan" or "captopril renal scintigraphy." Undoubtedly, this view of the action of angiotensin II and ACE inhibitors in the kidney with RAS is grossly oversimplified.

Majd et al. first reported the use of captopril to improve the diagnostic accuracy of scintigraphy in patients with underperfused kidneys.[78] His group later confirmed the usefulness of the test in a pediatric population, some of whom had coarctation of the aorta. A number of reports have followed (Table 6) and their variations in technique are apparent, as follows:

1. Different isotopes have been used. Although most groups that have compared the use of various isotopes have found DTPA to be most useful, Sfakianakis found this to be true of ^{131}I-iodohippurate.[83] Hovinga suggested that ^{99m}Tc-dimercaptosuccinic acid might be particularly useful in the diagnosis of segmental stenoses.[89]

2. Different criteria for a positive result have been used. Our group found that two parameters, used together, gave the best prediction of RVH:[86] (1) the ratio of glomerular filtration rate between the two kidneys greater than 1.5, and (2) the time to peak activity greater than or equal to 11 minutes. If either or both of these criteria were fulfilled, the test was labeled positive. The latter criterion was particularly helpful in identifying patients with bilateral stenoses and those with stenosis of the artery to a single kidney. Using these criteria, we achieved a sensitivity of 91% and a specificity of 93%. We feel that it is important that objective criteria such as these be used to determine whether a scan is positive. Some groups have included subjective changes in the shapes of the renogram curves in their criteria for positivity. This has the potential to introduce observer bias and render interpretation of the test by different observers less consistent.

3. Some investigators have required that patients discontinue all other medications for variable periods of time prior to taking the test. We feel that this may be dangerous and our results suggest that it is unnecessary. We allow our patients to take all medications other than ACE inhibitors up to and including the day of the scan. Lisinopril is withheld for 24 hours prior to the scan, enalapril is withheld for 12 hours, and, if the patient is on captopril, it is withheld on the morning of the scan only.

TABLE 6.
Previous Reports of Captopril Renal Scintigraphy*

Investigator	Reference	Number of Patients (RAS/total)	Radiopharmaceuticals	Captopril Dose and Duration	Preparation	Parameters Used for Positive Scan	Comments
Majd	78	8/14	DTPA	Variable		Deterioration of function post-captopril	"Dramatic" deterioration of function in all kidneys with RAS
Wenting	79	14/31	HIP Thal DTPA	150 mg/day × 3–5 weeks	All other medication withheld × 2 weeks	Not defined	Thal scan showed decreased filtration fraction in all cases; 50% of patients had decreased DTPA uptake; degree of stenosis not stated
Miyamori	80	8/20	HIP DTPA	37.5–75 mg/day × 1 week (repeated after 48 weeks)	Stopped all other anti-hypertensives × 2 weeks	Not defined	Fall in GFR post-captopril, $P < .01$
Geyskes	81	21/34 (15 cured by intervention)	HIP DTPA	25-mg single dose	Diuretics withheld × 2 days	DTPA uptake affected kidney/total <45%; difference in TIP >1 minute with HIP; 15-minute HIP activity affected/	Sensitivity 80%; specificity 100%

Study			Agent	Dose	Preparation	Criteria	Comments
Fommei	82	12/39†	DTPA	25-mg single dose	ACEI and diuretics withheld × 3 days	contralateral kidney ≥2.0; 2 of above 3 = positive result Decrease in GFR >25% following captopril	Sensitivity uncertain; not all patients had arteriograms
Sfakianakis	83	16/31	HIP DTPA	50-mg single dose	ACEI withheld 48 hours; other medications withheld overnight	HIP retention at 20 minutes <30% pre-captopril to >40% post-captopril	Not all controls had arteriograms; HIP more accurate than DTPA
Nally	84	11/16	HIP DTPA	25-mg single dose	ACEI withheld × 4 days; diuretics withheld 24–48 hours	Comparison between kidneys; maximum activity, delayed uptake, widening of peak activity, slow excretory phase	Subjective parameters; DTPA sensitivity 100%, specificity 100%
Pedersen	85	14/24	DTPA	24-mg single dose	8-hour fast, no fluids; subsequently given water mL/kg/hr; ACEI withheld × 2 weeks	Reduced single-kidney DTPA clearance >20%	Specificity 100%, sensitivity 100%
Chen	86	23/50	DTPA	50-mg single dose	ACEI withheld day of test only‡	TIP ≥11 minutes and/or GFR ratio between kidneys >1.5	Sensitivity 91%, specificity 93%

(Continued.)

TABLE 6 (cont.).

Investi-gator	Reference	Number of Patients (RAS/total)	Radiopharma-ceuticals	Captopril Dose and Duration	Preparation	Parameters Used for Positive Scan	Comments
						on pre- and/or post-captopril scans	
Svetkey	87	11/66	DTPA HIP	25-mg single dose	Beta-blockers and ACEI stopped × 2 weeks, diuretics × 48 hours; 4 g sodium per day diet	>6% difference between kidneys of GFR or ERPF	DTPA sensitivity 91%, specificity 50%; HIP sensitivity 80%, specificity 42%
Dondi	88	37/105	DTPA	50-mg single dose	Diuretics stopped × 48 hours; ACEI stopped × 1 week	>12% difference in kidney function; delayed TIP >5 minutes; or change in shape of renogram	Some criteria subjective; sensitivity 92%, specificity 97%
Hovinga	89	15/15	DTPA HIP	Enalapril 10 mg twice a day × 2 days	All medications stopped × 2 weeks	Flattening or lowering of curve	No control group; suggested DMSA may be useful in segmental stenosis

*ACEI = angiotensin-converting enzyme inhibitor; DMSA = ^{99m}Tc-dimercaptosuccinic acid; ERPF = effective renal plasma flow; DTPA = ^{99m}Tc-diethylenetriaminepentaacetic acid; GFR = glomerular filtration rate; HIP = ^{131}I-iodohippurate; RAS = renal artery stenosis; Thal = I-thalamate; TIP = time to peak activity.
†Includes two patients with coarctation. Note all 39 patients had arteriograms.
‡Lisinopril withheld the day before and the day of the test.

4. Some investigators have performed the baseline scan and the post-captopril scan on separate days. For convenience to the patient, however, it seems reasonable to perform the two arms of the test on the same day. The details of our protocol for simplified captopril scintigraphy are published elsewhere.[86]

Svetkey et al.[87] compared the usefulness of a variety of tests used to diagnose RVH. They found that captopril-stimulated peripheral PRA, with a sensitivity of 73% and a specificity of 72%, was superior to either scintigraphy or unstimulated renal vein renins. However, the negative predictive value of the captopril renogram in their hands was superior (96%, compared to 92% for stimulated peripheral PRA). Since the aim of any of these tests is to identify patients who do not require an arteriogram, this negative predictive value may be the most important determinant of the usefulness of the test.

The selection of patients for captopril scintigraphy, or for any method of diagnosing RVH, is of utmost importance. The sensitivity and specificity we obtained using the test (91% and 93%, respectively) were based on a population clinically selected as being at high risk of having the condition (see Table 2). Clearly, these figures would not be as favorable if the test were performed in an unselected group of hypertensives. We regard the test as a *case-finding* rather than a *screening* tool. It complements, rather than replaces, good clinical judgment.

Exercise renography

The hypothesis underlying the exercise renogram is that patients who have structural changes of the peripheral renal vasculature develop an exercise-induced disturbance in renal perfusion. These peripheral renal vascular changes render them surgically incurable. Conversely, in patients with potentially curable RVH, the renal perfusion is unaffected by exercise. This theory was tested by a German group using o-iodohippurate scintigraphy.[90] Out of ten patients with abnormal exercise renograms, nine failed to improve following technically successful surgery; out of eight patients with normal exercise renograms, surgery cured seven. These promising results support the aforementioned hypothesis. Further work on this test is clearly warranted.

This review has addressed the problems, and some of the solutions, in the diagnosis of RVH. The perfect solution to the problem has yet to be found but, in recent years, marked progress has been made, particularly in the scintigraphic methods of diagnosis. Our own approach to diagnosing the condition is as follows:

1. Identify which patients to investigate. A thorough history and physical examination is essential in this regard. As discussed previously, simple laboratory tests may be helpful also. One needs to identify at this stage the patients likely to have the disease in whom the benefit from a corrective

procedure (operative arterial reconstruction or angioplasty) probably outweighs the risk of investigation and management. Clearly, if a patient is not willing to go through with such a procedure, there is little point in pursuing the diagnosis.

2. We currently perform both captopril renal scintigraphy and digital renal arteriography. The arteriogram tells us whether RAS is present, but gives little information about the hemodynamic significance of a stenosis. There is some evidence to suggest that the captopril scintigram may provide useful information on the latter point.[91] In particular, should captopril convert a normal scintigram to abnormal or make an abnormal scan worse, curability after revascularization is much more likely.[92] However, we require more data before firm recommendations can be made regarding the value of captopril renal scintigraphy in this predictive role.

Picking out those patients with RVH from the whole population of hypertensives continues to be a challenging problem for clinicians. Significant new tools in our diagnostic armamentarium have been introduced in recent years to match the progress made in the treatment of the condition. A clear understanding of the pathophysiology of this disorder is important in selecting the procedures most worth investigating. The ideal test would be sensitive and specific, risk-free, inexpensive, and unaffected by concurrent medications. Further well-designed prospective studies are required to assess how closely our currently available tests approximate this ideal. Some of the recently introduced methods, such as captopril renal scintigraphy, appear to hold some promise. However, some of the other techniques have not withstood the test of time and it remains to be seen whether our initial enthusiasm for these radionuclide methods will be justified.

References

1. 1988 Joint National Committee: The 1988 report of the Joint National Committee on detection, evaluation and treatment of high blood pressure. *Arch Intern Med* 1988; 148:1023–1038.
2. Gifford RW Jr: Evaluation of the hypertensive patient with emphasis on detecting curable causes. *Milbank Q* 1969; 47:170–186.
3. Tucker RM, Labarthe DR: Frequency of surgical treatment for hypertension in adults at the Mayo Clinic from 1973 through 1975. *Mayo Clin Proc* 1979; 52:549–555.
4. Wilhelmson L, Berglund A: Prevalence of primary and secondary hypertension. *Am Heart J* 1977; 94:543–546.
5. Gifford RW Jr, Kirkendall W, O'Connor DT, et al: Office evaluation of hypertension. A statement for health professionals by a writing group of the Council for High Blood Pressure Research, American Heart Association. *Hypertension* 1989; 13:283–290.
6. Buxbaum M, Loibe U, Manker W, et al: *American Society of Nephrol 22nd Annual Meeting Proceedings* 1989; 209A.
7. Canzello VJ, Millan VA, Spiegel JE, et al: Percutaneous transluminal renal an-

gioplasty in management of atherosclerotic renovascular hypertension: Results in 100 patients. *Hypertension* 1989; 3:35–44.

8. Schreiber MJ, Pohl MA, Novick AC: The natural history of atherosclerotic and fibrous renal artery disease. *Urol Clin North Am* 1984; 11:383–392.
9. Wollenweber J, Sheps SG, David DG: Clinical course of atherosclerotic renovascular disease. *Am J Cardiol* 1968; 21:60–71.
10. Meaney TF, Dustan HP, McCormack LJ: Natural history of renal arterial disease. *Radiology* 1968; 9:877–887.
11. Holley KE, Hunt JC, Brown AL, et al: Renal artery stenosis. A clinical-pathologic study in normotensive and hypertensive patients. *Am J Med* 1964; 37:14.
12. Maxwell MH, Bleifer KH, Franklin SS, et al: Demographic analysis of the study. *JAMA* 1972; 220:1195–1204.
13. Maxwell MH, Kaufman JJ, Bleifer KH: Stenosing lesions of the renal arteries: Clinical manifestations. *Postgrad Med* 1966; 40:247–254.
14. Simon N, Franklin SS, Bleifer KH, et al: Clinical characteristics of renovascular hypertension. *JAMA* 1972; 220:1209–1218.
15. Anderson GH, Blakeman N, Streeten DHP: Prediction of renovascular hypertension. Comparison of clinical diagnostic indices. *Am J Hypertens* 1988; 1:301–304.
16. Messerli FH, Frohlich ED, Dreslinski GR, et al: Serum uric acid in essential hypertension: An indicator of renal vascular involvement. *Ann Intern Med* 1980; 93:817–821.
17. Tarazi RC, Frohlich ED, Dustan HP, et al: Hypertension and high hematocrit. Another clue to renal arterial disease. *Am J Cardiol* 1966; 18:855–858.
18. Kirchner JA, Kotchen TA, Galla JH, et al: Importance of chloride for acute inhibition of renin by sodium chloride. *Am J Physiol* 1978; 253:F444.
19. Laragh JH: Conceptual diagnostic and therapeutic dimensions of renin-system profiling of hypertensive disorders and of congestive heart failure: Your new research frontiers, in Doyle AE, Bearn AG (eds): *Hypertension and the Angiotensin System: Therapeutic Approaches.* New York, Raven Press, 1984, pp 47–72.
20. Ferrario CM, Schiavone MT: The renin angiotensin system: Importance in physiology and pathology. *Cleve Clin J Med* 1989; 56:439–446.
21. Rudnick MR, Maxwell MH: *Controversies in Nephrology and Hypertension.* New York, Churchill Livingstone, 1984.
22. Muller FB, Sealey JE, Case DB, et al: The captopril test for identifying renovascular disease in hypertensive patients. *Am J Med* 1986; 80:633–644.
23. Salvetti A, Arzilli F, Nuccorini A, et al: Does humoral and hemodynamic response to acute ACE inhibition identify true renovascular hypertension?, in Glorioso N (ed): *Renovascular Hypertension.* New York, Raven Press, 1987, pp 305–315.
24. Idrissi A, Fournier A, Renaud H, et al: The captopril challenge test as a screening test for renovascular hypertension. *Kidney Int* 1988; 34(suppl 25):S138–S141.
25. Derkx FHM, Tan-Tjiong HL, Wenting GJ, et al: Captopril test for diagnosis of renal artery stenosis, in Glorioso N (ed): *Renovascular Hypertension.* New York, Raven Press, 1987, pp 295–304.
26. Postma CT, Van der Steen PH, Hoefnagels WH, et al: The captopril test in the detection of renovascular disease in hypertensive patients. *Arch Intern Med* 1990; 150:625–628.

27. Frederickson ED, Wilcox CS, Bucci CM, et al: A prospective evaluation of a simplified captopril test for the detection of renovascular hypertension. *Arch Intern Med* 1990; 150:569–572.
28. Marks LS, Maxwell MH, Smith RB, et al: Detection of renovascular hypertension: Saralasin test versus renin determinations. *J Urol* 1976; 116:406–409.
29. Webb DJ, Cumming AMM, Adams FC, et al: Changes in active and inactive renin and in angiotensin II across the kidney in essential hypertension and renal artery stenosis. *J Hypertens* 1984; 2:605.
30. Maxwell MH, Marks LS, Lupu AN, et al: Predictive value of renin determinations in renal artery stenosis. *JAMA* 1977; 238:2617–2620.
31. Kaplan NM: Renal vascular hypertension, in *Clinical Hypertension,* ed 4. Baltimore, Williams & Wilkins, 1986, pp 317–344.
32. Morlin C, Torelius LE, Wide L: Spontaneous variations in renal vein renin activity in man. *Clin Chim Acta* 1982; 119:31.
33. Vaughan ED Jr, Buhler FR, Laragh JH, et al: Renovascular hypertension: Renin measurements to indicate hypersecretion and contralateral suppression, estimate renal plasma flow and score for surgical curability. *Am J Med* 1973; 55:402.
34. Couch NP, Sullivan J, Crane C: The predictive accuracy of renal vein renin activity in the surgery of renovascular hypertension. *Surgery* 1976; 79:70–76.
35. Melman A, Donohue JP, Weinberger MH, et al: Improved diagnostic accuracy of renal venous renin ratios with stimulation of renin release. *J Urol* 1977; 117:145.
36. Strong CG, Hunt JC, Sheps SG, et al: Renal venous renin activity. Enhancement of sensitivity of lateralization by sodium depletion. *Am J Cardiol* 1971; 27:602–611.
37. Thind GS, Montojo PM, Johnson A, et al: Enhancement of renal venous renin ratios by intravenous hydralazine in renovascular hypertension. *Am J Cardiol* 1984; 53:109–115.
38. Stokes GS, Weber MA, Gain J, et al: Diazoxide-induced renin release in diagnosis of remediable renovascular hypertension. *Aust N Z J Med* 1976; 6:26–29.
39. Re R, Novelline R, Escourrou M-T, et al: Inhibition of angiotensin-converting enzyme for diagnosis of renal-artery stenosis. *N Engl J Med* 1978; 298:582–586.
40. Thibonnier M, Joseph A, Sassano P, et al: Improved diagnosis of unilateral renal artery lesions after captopril administration. *JAMA* 1984; 251:56–60.
41. Lyons DF, Streck WF, Kem DC, et al: Captopril stimulation of differential renins in renovascular hypertension. *Hypertension* 1983; 5:615–622.
42. Rosenthal T, Morag B, Holtzman E, et al: Use of oral converting enzyme inhibitor, captopril for lateralizing renal venous renin activity. *Clin Exp Hypertens [A]* 1983; A5:1629–1634.
43. Morganti A, Gammaro L, Sala C, et al: Effects of acute converting enzyme inhibition and renal angioplasty on active and inactive renin and angiotensin II in the renal veins of patients with renovascular hypertension: A preliminary report, in Glorioso N (eds): *Renovascular Hypertension.* Raven Press, New York, 1987, pp 383–397.
44. Stamey TA, Nudelman IJ, Good PH, et al: Functional characteristics of renovascular hypertension. *Medicine* 1961; 40:347.
45. Howard JE, Connor TB: Hypertension produced by unilateral renal disease. *Arch Intern Med* 1962; 109:8.

46. Dean RH, Foster JH: Criteria for the diagnosis of renovascular hypertension. *Surgery* 1973; 74:926–930.
47. Boughton RM, Sommers SC: A new concept of renal hypertension. *J Urol* 1963; 89:133–136.
48. Crocker DW, Newton RA, Mahoney EM, et al: Hypertension due to primary renal ischemia: A correlation of juxtaglomerular cell counts with clinicopathological findings in twenty-five cases. *N Engl J Med* 1962; 267:794–800.
49. Cigarroa RG, Lange RA, Williams RH, et al: Dosing of contrast material to prevent contrast nephropathy in patients with renal disease. *Am J Med* 1989; 86:649–652.
50. Schwab SJ, Hlatky MA, Pieper KS, et al: Contrast nephrotoxicity: A randomized controlled trial of a nonionic and an ionic radiographic contrast agent. *N Engl J Med* 1989; 320:149–153.
51. Aron NB, Feinfeld DA, Peters AT, et al: Acute renal failure associated with ioxaglate, a low-osmolality radiocontrast agent. *Am J Kidney Dis* 1989; 13:189–193.
52. Parfrey PS, Griffiths SM, Barrett BJ, et al: Contrast material-induced renal failure in patients with diabetes mellitus, renal insufficiency, or both. A prospective controlled study. *N Engl J Med* 1989; 320:143–149.
53. Bakris GL, Burnett JC: A role for calcium in radiocontrast-induced reductions in renal hemodynamics. *Kidney Int* 1985; 27:465–468.
54. Zabbo A, Novick AC: Digital subtraction angiography for noninvasive imaging of the renal artery. *Urol Clin North Am* 1984; 11:409–416.
55. Havey RJ, Krumlovsky F, delGreco F, et al: Screening for renovascular hypertension. Is renal digital-subtraction angiography the preferred noninvasive test? *JAMA* 1985; 254:388–392.
56. Smith CW, Winfield AC, Price RR, et al: Evaluation of digital venous angiography for the diagnosis of renovascular hypertension. *Radiology* 1982; 144:51–54.
57. Correa RJ, Stewart BH, Boblitt DF: Intravenous pyelography as a screening test in renal hypertension. *Am J Roentgenol* 1962; 88:1135–1141.
58. Maxwell MH, Gonick HC, Wiita R, et al: Use of the rapid-sequence intravenous pyelogram in the diagnosis of renovascular hypertension. *N Engl J Med* 1964; 270:213–220.
59. Bookstein JJ, Abrams HL, Buenger RE, et al: Radiological aspects of renovascular hypertension. Part 2. The role of urography in unilateral renovascular disease. *JAMA* 1972; 220:1225–1230.
60. Bookstein JJ, Abrams HL, Buenger RE, et al: Radiologic aspects of renovascular hypertension. 2. The role of urography in unilateral renovascular disease. *JAMA* 1972; 220:1225–1230.
61. Bookstein JJ, Maxwell MH, Abrams HL, et al: Cooperative study of radiologic aspects of renovascular hypertension. Bilateral renovascular disease. *JAMA* 1977; 237:1706–1709.
62. Thornbury JR, Stanley JC, Fryback DG: Hypertensive urogram: A nondiscriminatory test for renovascular hypertension. *AJR* 1982; 138:43–46.
63. Lewis BD, James EM: Current applications of duplex and color Doppler ultrasound imaging: Abdomen. *Mayo Clin Proc* 1989; 64:1158–1169.
64. Avasthi PS, Voyles WF, Greene ER: Noninvasive diagnosis of renal artery stenosis by echo-Doppler velocimetry. *Kidney Int* 1984; 25:824–829.
65. Norris CS, Pfeiffer JS, Rittgers SE, et al: Noninvasive evaluation of renal artery stenosis and renovascular resistance. Experimental and clinical studies. *J Vasc Surg* 1984; 1:192–201.

66. Kohler TR, Zierler RE, Martin RL, et al: Noninvasive diagnosis of renal artery stenosis by ultrasonic duplex scanning. *J Vasc Surg* 1986; 4:450–456.
67. Taylor DC, Kettler MD, Moneta GL, et al: Duplex ultrasound scanning in the diagnosis of renal artery stenosis: A prospective evaluation. *J Vasc Surg* 1988; 7:363–369.
68. Strandness DE: Duplex scanning in the diagnosis of renovascular hypertension. *Surg Clin North Am* 1990; 70:109–116.
69. Greene ER, Avasthi PS, Hodges JW: Noninvasive Doppler assessment of renal artery stenosis and hemodynamics. *J Clin Ultrasound* 1987; 15:653–659.
70. Taylor KJW, Morse SS, Rigsby CM, et al: Vascular complications in renal allografts: Detection with duplex Doppler US. *Radiology* 1987; 162:31–38.
71. Maxwell M: Cooperative study of renovascular hypertension: Current status. *Kidney Int* 1975; 8(suppl):153–160.
72. Chiarini C, Esposti ED, Iosinno F, et al: Renal scintigraphy versus renal vein renin activity for identifying and treating renovascular hypertension. *Nephron* 1982; 32:8–13.
73. Gross ML, Nally JV, Windham JP, et al: Improved computer-assisted nuclear imaging in renovascular hypertension. *J Clin Hypertens* 1985; 4:326–335.
74. Mantero F, Fallo F, Scarone C, et al: Radioisotopic studies in renovascular hypertension before and after surgery or percutaneous transluminal renal angioplasty, in Glorioso N (eds): *Renovascular Hypertension.* Raven Press, New York, 1987, pp 425–430.
75. Reid IA: The renin-angiotensin system and body function. *Arch Intern Med* 1985; 145:1475.
76. Edwards RM: Segmental effects of norepinephrine and angiotensin II on isolated renal microvessels. *Am J Physiol* 1983; 244:F526.
77. Nally JV: The captopril tests: A new concept in detecting renovascular hypertension? *Cleve Clin J Med* 1989; 56:395–401.
78. Majd M, Potter BM, Guzzetta PC, et al: Captopril enhanced renal scintigraphy for detection of renal artery stenosis—an update. *J Nucl Med* 1986; 27-II:962.
79. Wenting GJ, Tan-Tjiong HL, Derkx FHM, et al: Split renal function after captopril in unilateral renal artery stenosis. *Br Med J [Clin Res]* 1984; 288:886–890.
80. Miyamori I, Yasuhara S, Takeda Y, et al: Effects of converting enzyme inhibition on split renal function in renovascular hypertension. *Hypertension* 1986; 8:415–421.
81. Geyskes GG, Oei HY, Puylaert BAJ, et al: Renovascular hypertension identified by captopril-induced changes in the renogram. *Hypertension* 1987; 9:451–458.
82. Fommei E, Ghione S, Palla L, et al: Renal scintigraphic captopril test in the diagnosis of renovascular hypertension. *Hypertension* 1987; 10:212–220.
83. Sfakianakis GN, Jaffe DJ, Bourgoignie JJ: Captopril scintigraphy in the diagnosis of renovascular hypertension. *Kidney Int* 1988; 34:S142–S144.
84. Nally JV, Gupta BK, Clarke HS, et al: Captopril renography for the detection of renovascular hypertension. *Cleve Clin J Med* 1988; 55:311–318.
85. Pedersen EB, Jensen FT, Eiskjoer H, et al: Differentiation between renovascular and essential hypertension by means of changes in single kidney 99mTc-DTPA clearance induced by angiotensin-converting enzyme inhibition. *Am J Hypertens* 1989; 2:323–334.
86. Chen CC, Hoffer PB, Vahjen G: A simple method of Tc-99mDTPA captopril renal scintigraphy analysis in patients at high risk for renal artery stenosis. *Radiology* 1990; 176:365–370.

87. Svetkey LP, Himmelstein SI, Dunnick NR, et al: Prospective analysis of strategies for diagnosing renovascular hypertension. *Hypertension* 1989; 14:247–257.

88. Dondi M, Franchi R, Levorato M, et al: Evaluation of hypertensive patients by means of captopril enhanced renal scintigraphy with Technecium 99m DTPA. *J Nucl Med* 1989; 30:615–621.

89. Hovinga TKK, deJong PE, Piers DA, et al: Diagnostic use of angiotensin converting enzyme inhibitors in radioisotope evaluation of unilateral renal artery stenosis. *J Nucl Med* 1989; 30:605–614.

90. Clorius JH, Allenberg J, Hupp T, et al: Predictive value of exercise renography for presurgical evaluation of nephrogenic hypertension. *Hypertension* 1987; 10:280–286.

91. Setaro JF, Roer DA, Meier GH, et al: Use of simplified captopril renal scintigraphy in prediction of outcome with renal artery revascularization. *Circulation* 1989; 80(suppl II):II–21.

92. Meier GH, Sumpio B, Black HR, et al: Captopril renal scintigraphy—an advance in the detection and treatment of renovascular hypertension? *J Vasc Surg* 1990; 11:770–777.

Advances in Genitourinary Laparoscopy

David A. Bloom, M.D.

Associate Professor of Surgery, University of Michigan Medical School; Chief, Pediatric Urology, Mott Children's Hospital, Ann Arbor, Michigan

Kurt Semm, o. Prof. Dr. Med Dr. Med. Vet h.c.

Direktor der Abteilung Frauenheilkunde im Klinikum der Christian-Albrechts-Universität, Kiel, Germany

I believe it will scarcely be denied that one of the most important characteristics and improvements of modern medicine consists in the direct exploration of organs. . . . Agreeably to the old adage that 'Naught is new under the sun,' as each addition to our means of diagnosis has been brought under the notice of our profession, claimants have sprung up to dispute the honor and credit of invention.[1]

F.R. Cruise, 1865

The Background

In 1865, when practical cystoscopy was still a dream, Francis Richard Cruise, medical officer at the Mater Misericordiae Hospital in Dublin, looked beyond the obvious urinary tract applications of his homemade cystoscope and suggested that this instrument might someday permit direct visual inspection of *any* body cavity.[1] Forty-five years later in Stockholm, Hans Christian Jacobeus, professor of medicine at the Karolinska Institute, became the first to apply a cystoscope beyond the genitourinary tracts. He developed techniques for thoracoscopy and laparoscopy in cadavers and extended the procedure to living patients.[2] His sequence of steps for diagnostic laparoscopy is astonishing in its similarity to present methods. Laparoscopy subsequently found its main applications in gynecologic practice. In 1934 Werner used high-frequency current via laparotomy for tubal sterilization, and in 1936 Bosch applied the technique through a laparoscope.[3, 4] Palmer described a method for ovarian biopsy through a laparoscope in 1946.[5] Today, Semm's instruments and techniques for intraperitoneal endoscopic surgical maneuvers take laparoscopy far beyond simple clip application, cauterization, and biopsy.[6] It is no longer completely accurate to describe these techniques as *laparoscopy; lapara,* the Greek term for flank,

Reprinted from *Advances in Urology,*® vol. 4.
Copyright 1991, Mosby–Year Book, Inc.

has somewhat carelessly become synonymous with *abdomen.* Celioscopy or peritoneoscopy are better descriptions of general intra-abdominal endoscopy, and pelviscopy is perhaps the most accurate term for examination of the pelvic viscera including the bladder, internal genital structures, and inguinal canals. Although laparoscopy is the most widely used term for intra-abdominal and pelvic endoscopy, accurate usage would prefer celiopelviscopy.

Urological interest in celiopelviscopy remained restrained. In 1976, Cortesi's group from the departments of surgery and endocrinology at the University of Modena was the first to describe endoscopic localization of nonpalpable testes: bilateral abdominal testes were identified by laparoscope in an 18-year-old and this technique was commended to urologists as a prelude to surgical exploration in the management of patients with nonpalpable gonads.[7] Paramo's experience in Madrid with laparoscopy in six men during the years 1975 to 1977 was belatedly described in a letter to the *Journal of Urology.*[8] Silber, in 1980, reported laparoscopy in three males, including one child.[9] In 1982, Scott, at Newcastle-upon-Tyne, authored the first pediatric laparoscopy series consisting of 14 boys with nonpalpable testes.[10] In spite of subsequent reports, laparoscopy is still not standard practice in managing children with nonpalpable testes (Table 1).[10–19] Celiopelviscopy is a useful first operative step for children with nonpalpable testes and it obviates extensive preoperative investigations. In addition, Semm's methods introduce a number of additional endoscopic procedures into the genitourinary armamentarium.

The Technique of Celiopelviscopy

Anesthetic concerns are of paramount importance during celiopelviscopy. Pulse oximeters are standard practice with most pediatric general anesthet-

TABLE 1.
Laparoscopy for Nonpalpable Testes: Major Reports

Author	Year	Number of Patients	Reference
Scott	1982	14	10
Lowe et al.	1984	33	11
Malone & Guiney	1984	38	12
Boddy et al.	1985	46	13
Manson et al.	1985	14	14
Weiss & Seashore	1987	32	15
Bloom et al.	1988	28	16
Das & Amar	1988	16	17
Naslund et al.	1989	21	18
Guiney et al.	1989	86	19

ics and should not be omitted during celiopelviscopy. End-tidal CO_2 monitoring is important to detect CO_2 absorption and may be a clue to gas embolus. Although high regional anesthetics are acceptable for pelviscopy, we prefer general anesthesia in children (with back-up caudal blocks when concomitant open surgery is anticipated). With general anesthetics, patients undergo endotracheal intubation because of the possibility of regurgitation. The stomach is emptied to obviate the chance of gastric puncture. Some anesthesiologists avoid the use of nitrous oxide with pelviscopy for fear of feeding a gas embolus, but this has not been deemed a practical concern at our center. Muscle relaxants minimize the chance for bucking and bowel injury. Additionally, abdominal wall muscle rigidity in concert with a pneumoperitoneum can create enough pressure to lead to catastrophic impairment of venous return at the cardiac level.

After induction of anesthesia, the bladder is decompressed with a small catheter and the table is turned to place the patient with a moderate reverse Trendelenburg (15-degree head-down) tilt. The umbilicus (which often contains enough topsoil for a small garden in young boys) is prepped with a povidone solution on a cotton-tipped applicator. After palpation of the aorta and its bifurcation, a Veress pneumoperitoneum cannula is placed in the umbilicus, pointed at the sacral promontory, and punctured into the peritoneal cavity. At this point, we establish proper needle position first by moving it from side to side to check its mobility and next by injecting a small amount of saline through it. The saline should inject easily, but cannot be aspirated back when the needle is in the intraperitoneal space. The valve to the insufflator is opened and the abdomen is distended with CO_2 at pressures less than 12 mm Hg. The pneumoperitoneum is gauged visibly and by percussion. Percussion of gas over the liver is good evidence of intraperitoneal inflation. During filling, one must palpate the distended abdomen frequently and examine the insufflator pressure gauge to prevent overdistention. Once a satisfactory pneumoperitoneum (10 to 12 mm Hg) is established, we make a small infraumbilical skin incision. A 5-mm endoscopic sheath with conical-tip trocar is inserted through the incision in a z-shaped pathway. The trocar is replaced by the 30-degree lens. Low-pressure automatic continuous insufflation maintains satisfactory visibility for the duration of the examination. Nonetheless, one must reassess the degree of distention continuously by both palpation and pressure gauge. A second puncture is sometimes necessary for a probe or other instrument to move omentum or a loop of bowel that obscures the field of vision. This is done by directing the pelviscope toward the suprapubic region and making a small stab wound in the midline over the lighted area. A trocar is passed through the stab wound and twisted into the distended peritoneal cavity under direct pelviscopic vision. Additional suprapubic puncture sites are made for additional instruments as necessary in lateral suprapublic sites, utilizing a z-shaped path and taking care to avoid the epigastric vessels. When open exploration follows laparoscopy, we reprepare and drape the field to assure complete aseptic technique.

Complications of celiopelviscopy are minimized by a strict set of safety steps. First, one must be familiar with the operation of the insufflator and have an adequate supply of CO_2. The spring-action and flow through the Veress needle are checked and we assure that anesthesia and relaxation are satisfactory before making the puncture. The Veress needle is grasped firmly at the hub so that the blunt obturator protrudes in the resting position. The puncture should be clean and quick through the preperitoneal space and into the peritoneal cavity, stopping short of retroperitoneum. The flow is turned off during puncture to prevent insufflation of the preperitoneal space during transit of the needle. Needle mobility and an injection/aspiration test are checked prior to insufflation. Throughout the diagnostic and interventional endoscopic steps we keep an eye on the intraperitoneal pressure, a hand on the abdomen, and an ear to the anesthesiologist. At the conclusion of celiopelviscopy the gas is decompressed, the instruments are removed, and the stab wounds are closed with subcuticular absorbable synthetic sutures. A list of potential complications includes abdominal wall hemorrhage, preperitoneal emphysema, visceral puncture, omental laceration, omental evisceration, large vessel injury, gas embolus, CO_2 absorption, overdistention, arrhythmia, cardiac arrest, wound infection, and peritonitis. Most complications are related to the creation of the pneumoperitoneum.[20] In gynecologic laparoscopy, high-frequency electrical current is responsible for many visceral injuries.[6] There is a learning

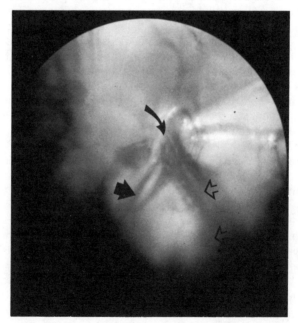

FIG 1.
Normal anatomy at the right internal inguinal ring. The *curved arrow* indicates the internal ring, the *open arrow* indicates the spermatic vessels, and the *wide arrow* indicates the vas deferens.

curve with the laparoscope, but careful training and deliberate technique make this a safe procedure.

The normal pelviscopic anatomic field in males is outlined by the bladder with its ligaments anteriorly, the internal inguinal rings laterally, and the rectum posteriorly. The vas deferens passes over the obliterated umbilical artery and then sweeps caudally to disappear into the internal inguinal ring. The spermatic vessels enter the internal ring from the inferolateral aspect (Fig 1). Small bowel and appendix may cover spermatic vessels on the right, whereas descending and sigmoid colon is more likely to obscure the landmarks at the left internal ring. Ureters are medial and inferior to the spermatic vessels, and are usually more difficult to find. Abnormal pelviscopic findings include supracanalicular gonad, blind-ending spermatic vessels, absent vas deferens, inguinal hernia, or single umbilical ligament. Persistent müllerian structures, namely uterus, fallopian tube, or proximal vagina, are rare, but potential findings. This situation, once known as hernia uteri inguinalis, occurs when these structures are found in genetic males, the suspected cause being failure to elaborate müllerian inhibitory subtance.[21]

The Nonpalpable Testis

Nonpalpable testes comprise only a small part of the spectrum of abnormalities of testicular descent and the wide range of reported incidences[22] is influenced by referral pattern and skill in examination. Incidences reported include 20% by Jones, 12% by Scorer, and 8% by Betran-Brown and Villegas-Alvarez.[23-25] Jackson et al. found that 13% of undescended testes were impalpable under anesthesia.[26] It is generally easier to examine testes in an awake child, as long as he is relaxed and cooperative. A little time spent gaining rapport is a worthwhile investment. We initiate examination over the area of the internal inguinal ring and gently walk our fingers distally down the canal toward the scrotum. This may be repeated a few times, and if a gonad has not been felt, we place water-soluble lubricant over the skin to improve tactile perception. Lymph nodes are usually a bit more superficial, lateral, and firm than testes. When supine examination fails to elicit the testis, examination in a cross-leg sitting posture may be more successful. Only after very diligent examinations will we declare a testis nonpalpable.

Nonpalpable testes pose some clinical dilemmas. In a child, the potential of an occult testis is compromised because of its abnormal location. For an adult, an occult testis is a liability, not only because it is more susceptible to malignancy.[27] but also because early detection of malignancy by self-examination is not possible. A nonpalpable testis must be located or its absence confirmed. Definition of absence requires the observation of blind-ending spermatic vessels; a blind-ending vas by itself is not sufficient proof of absence.[28] If a testis is located in an extrascrotal position, it needs to be moved or removed. Inguinal exploration and intraperitoneal inspection are the traditional means of diagnosis: when inguinal exploration fails to reveal a testis or prove its absence, the incision is extended or an alternate incision is made to look above the internal ring from an intraperitoneal vantage. With the hope of facilitating or obviating surgery, each new imaging modality, in its turn, has been applied to nonpalpable testes: arteriography, venography, herniography, computerized tomography, and ultrasonography all have been evaluated, but none of these has been reliable in locating a testis or confirming its absence.[29–33] Magnetic resonance imaging provides nice gonadal detail and may be advantageous over the older methods.[34] Hinman in one report, and Gearhart and Jeffs in another, reviewed localization modalities and found no reliable substitute for surgical exploration.[35, 36] The mission of the urologist extends beyond localization or identification of absence; even if a technique proved completely accurate and reliable in locating a testis or defining absence, we believe something further needs to be done surgically on most patients.

Celiopelviscopy for Nonpalpable Testes

Our approach to a boy with a nonpalpable testis begins with the endoscope. The goal is to visually locate an occult testis or prove its absence by finding blind-ending spermatic vessels and vas deferens. The primary focus of pelviscopic attention is the internal inguinal ring (see Fig 1) and subsequent operative steps are determined by the findings at that site.

Normal Anatomy and Variants at the Internal Inguinal Ring.— When normal anatomy is identified at the internal ring (that is, when the vas and spermatic vessels pass into the ring), it is likely that a testis transited this site at some earlier point in time. Normal pelviscopic anatomy at the internal ring justifies distal exploration, this being open inguinal exploration. In one group of boys, we find a distal gonad that was missed on physical examination; these are usually hypoplastic testes. The distal gonad is managed by orchiopexy or orchiectomy as dictated by the clinical situation. In the other main subset of boys, inguinal exploration fails to find a testis. There may be a blind-ending sac or other remnant, or there may be no cord structures distal to the internal ring. Because we have identified normal anatomy at the internal ring, we assume the testis was lost from prior vascular accident, in all probability this was antenatal or perinatal torsion of the spermatic cord. Agenesis of the testis is an unlikely explanation and probably would require the presence of some ipsilateral müllerian structures (which would have been seen at pelviscopy). The primary value of laparoscopy in these instances is that there is no need to go beyond an inguinal exploration if neither gonad nor blind-ending cord structures are seen, because pelviscopy already has established proximal cord structures.

Weiss first recognized that the presence of a patent processus vaginalis at the internal ring is evidence for a more distal gonad (Fig 2).[15] On occasions we have observed an abrupt transition from a normal thick vascular leash to a very hypoplastic string of spermatic vessels entering the internal

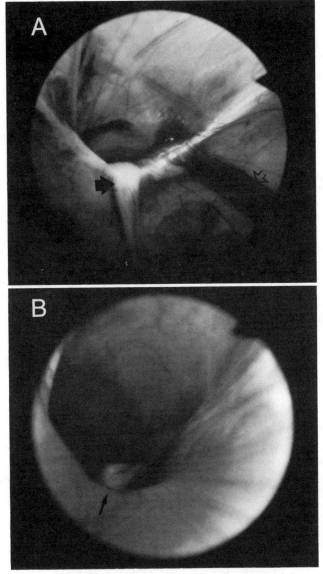

FIG 2.
A, patent right processus vaginalis (inguinal hernia) at internal ring. The *open arrow* indicates the spermatic vessels, and the *wide arrow* indicates the vas deferens. **B,** view inside patent right processus vaginalis. The *arrow* indicates the small testis in the midinguinal canal.

ring. In most of these instances, no distal gonad is found on the subsequent inguinal exploration and it may be reasonable to defer inguinal exploration if the spermatic vessels at the internal ring are markedly hypoplastic or atretic.

The Supracanalicular Testis.—In some boys with nonpalpable testes, celiopelviscopy locates a high gonad at, or proximal to, the internal inguinal ring (Fig 3). Although we describe these as "intra-abdominal," we recognize that such gonads are truly retroperitoneal, lying behind the thin peritoneal membrane, but they are best seen from within the peritoneum just as the ovary is best located from this vantage. Surgical choices depend upon the clinical situation. Hinman challenges that salvage of a unilateral high testis may not be desirable: "An undercurrent of opinion runs that if the contralateral testis is normal . . . taxing surgical maneuvers are not warranted and orchiectomy is the more sensible course.[35] In a postpubertal male with a small intra-abdominal testis and a normal contralateral testis, the usual choice is orchiectomy. With knowledge of the exact location of the testis, access to it is simplified and a small incision is made directly over it. Another option is endoscopic removal of the testis. Endoscopic oophorectomy with Semm's operative endoscopic instruments and techniques is safe and practical, and there is no reason why this cannot be extended to the testis.

In some circumstances, efforts to save a high testis are warranted; in younger boys or cases of bilaterality, the high testis may be worth an attempt at salvage. Testes just at the internal ring sometimes can be brought down into the scrotum by simple orchiopexy techniques. Abdominal testes in boys with prune belly syndrome usually can be brought into the scrotum

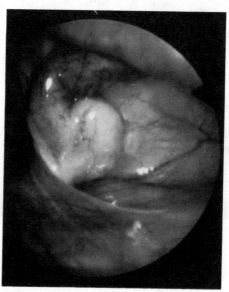

FIG 3.
Left internal inguinal ring with testis just proximal to it.

in the first year of life. This may appear impossible at first, but after the spermatic vessel leash is freed from the tortuous ureters, enough mobility will be available for simple orchiopexy. One usually can judge the length and potential of the spermatic vessels during pelviscopy and make a fair judgment regarding amenability to routine orchiopexy.

When the vascular leash is inadequate, options include staged orchiopexy, Fowler-Stephens orchiopexy, or microvascular autotransplantation.[37, 39] The standard approach to the high testis was defined in 1959 by Fowler and Stephens. They described paraepididymal anastomoses between internal spermatic and vasal arteries in some patients with a nonpalpable testis, a short internal spermatic vascular plexus, and a long loop of vas deferens.[38] Such testes may remain adequately vascularized by their vasal collaterals after ligation and division of the spermatic vascular leash. Among the preconditions for a successful outcome from this operation, the long loop anomaly must be present, the peritesticular anastomoses must be preserved, and testicular infarction must be prevented. Even if all preconditions are met, the long-loop orchiopexy with spermatic vessel division may result in testicular loss. Duckett, in 1982, advocated in situ spermatic vessel ligation followed by staged Fowler-Stephens orchiopexy,[40] and in 1984 Ransley et al. reported on this.[41] Celiopelviscopy permits a new twist to these approaches, namely staging Fowler-Stephens orchiopexy with clip ligation of the spermatic vessels.[16] A Hulka clip is placed high on the spermatic vascular leash at the time of pelviscopy to augment the vasal collateral blood supply and 6 months later the patient undergoes Fowler-Stephens orchiopexy. Rajfer's group showed that collateral augmentation occurs in rats within 30 days of spermatic vessel interruption.[42]

The Solitary Testis.—The majority of instances of congenital monorchia involve a missing left testis.[28, 43] In the absence of müllerian remnants on that side, the presumption is that a testis must have been present in the first two trimesters to produce müllerian inhibitory substance. Late gestation or perinatal loss of the testis may be due to some specific vulnerability of the left-sided vascular supply. Whatever the cause, the missing testis cannot be brought back. A normal contralateral testis usually will be adequate for hormonal and reproductive function, but as Harris wrote, "When a child is found to have only one testis, that gonad assumes a value beyond all measure."[44] Its loss is a catastrophe. The main risks to the testis during childhood are trauma and torsion. After childhood, an added concern is neoplasia. Families and patients must be counseled regarding protection of the testis during contact sports, self-examination, and the need to seek urgent medical attention for testicular pain or swelling. Furthermore, we agree with Harris in advocating prophylactic fixation of a solitary testis at the same time as pelviscopy. Whereas no form of testicular fixation can guarantee against subsequent torsion, most methods should minimize the odds. The important point is that the testis must be anchored, but not damaged. Fixation orchiopexy is unlikely to cause any harm if a nonreactive suture material is employed (we prefer Vicryl) and if sutures do not disturb the integrity of the tunica albuginea.[45]

Male Pelviscopy at the University of Michigan

Celiopelviscopy on the urology service at the University of Michigan is evolving from a purely diagnostic to an interventional procedure. We initially employed the laparoscope diagnostically in a boy who was referred after a negative inguinal exploration for a nonpalpable testis. This was suspected to be an instance of blind-ending spermatic vessels and vas, presumably secondary to old torsion, but proof of absence (in that exploration was not carried to the point to demonstrate the blind-ending vessels) was incomplete. We thought that pelviscopy would spare him the need for another incision. This was indeed the situation, and we followed the lead of others (see Table 1) in instituting celiopelviscopy as our first operative maneuver in boys with nonpalpable testes. This was carried a step further when we began to stage Fowler-Stephens orchiopexy by means of Hulka clip application in selected patients. The clip also seemed a logical way to perform varicocele ligation. The next logical step will be endoscopic orchiectomy.

Our pelviscopy series in boys consists of 77 patients aged 6 months to 41 years. Seventy-six patients had nonpalpable testes and 1 had a varicocele. Among the 76 patients, 37 had a nonpalpable left testis, 28 had a nonpalpable right testis, and the problem was bilateral in 11 (Table 2). Therefore, there were 87 nonpalpable testes. The patients fell into three main groups in addition to a few with unusual findings.

In one group of patients, testes were seen intra-abdominally, above the internal inguinal ring. Among 22 patients, the abdominal testes were bilateral in 5, right-sided in 10, and left-sided in 7. We utilized a variation of staged orchiopexy with endoscopic placement of a Hulka clip in 10 patients. Nine of these have come to orchiopexy. In 1, who had undergone previous inguinal-only exploration, the testis was atrophic. The other 8

TABLE 2.
Laparoscopy for Nonpalpable Testes

Clinical Finding	Number of Patients	Right	Left	Bilateral
Blind vessels	30	9	19	2
Missed low testes	19	8	7	4
Abdominal testes	22	10	7	5
Absent vessels	4	0	4	0
Transverses testicular ectopia (TTE)	1	1	0	0
Total	76	28	37	11

have viable testes that survived both the clip placement and the subsequent Fowler-Stephens long-loop orchiopexy without loss of testicular size.

The second group of 30 patients had normal anatomy at the internal inguinal ring or vas and vessels ending proximal to the ring. Inguinal exploration revealed a cord remnant or empty canal and a diagnosis of blind vessels was made. These patients presumably had loss of the testis from prior vascular accident. The absent testis was bilateral in 2 instances and left-sided in 19 (68%), a predisposition described by others.[28, 43] In some patients, the spermatic vessels leading down to the internal ring were appreciably hypoplastic, whereas in others they were unremarkable. The contralateral testes are usually normal and we anchored these in the scrotum to minimize the opportunity for subsequent torsion.

The third group also had normal anatomy at the internal ring, but inguinal exploration revealed testes in the inguinal canal or superficial pouch that had been missed in spite of careful preoperative physical examination. These gonads were usually hypoplastic. Of the 19 patients, 4 had bilateral missed low testes and the unilateral instances were divided nearly evenly between right (8) and left (7). The smallness and frequent bilaterality of these missed low testes suggests an underlying endocrinopathy.

A few unusual findings merit comment. In 4 patients, all with a left nonpalpable testis, we failed to see either a high testis or any evidence of spermatic vessels at the internal ring. No müllerian structures were visible through the endoscope. We explored the retroperitoneum in 3 of these boys, but found no testes. In 1 such patient, an atretic strand of spermatic vessels led down to the internal ring. Although we could see this on direct inspection from the retroperitoneal side of the peritoneal membrane, it had not been visible through the laparoscope. In the other 2 patients, we could not identify spermatic vessels. A fourth patient, with ultrasonographic renal agenesis on the side of the nonpalpable testis, had neither vessels, vas, nor gonad visible endoscopically and underwent no further investigation or exploration. Therefore, in 3 of 76 patients, laparoscopy did not prevent diagnostic open exploration above the canal. The patient with the vascular remnant possibly should be reassigned to the blind-vessel group. The explanation for the remaining 2 patients is difficult: one cannot easily make a diagnosis of testicular agenesis in the absence of ipsilateral müllerian structures. We suspect, even in the 2 patients without a visible spermatic vascular remnant, that there must have been a gonad in the first two trimesters of intrauterine life and that it subsequently was lost through some vascular accident.

Three other extraordinary situations merit comment. A 41-year-old man was found to have a nonpalpable gonad on a physical examination required before joining a military reserve unit. His contralateral testis was normal and there was no history of trauma or symptoms of scrotal pain or swelling. We discussed the options of imaging studies, surgical exploration, laparoscopy, or doing nothing. Although he was just past the usual age range for most testicular tumors, we felt that a recommendation for no further evaluation or treatment would carry a tacit guarantee that an occult gonad would cause him no harm. We did not believe that any imaging studies could definitively prove absence. Furthermore, if imaging studies located a testis, we would remove it. We recommended celiopelviscopy. A small "intra-abdominal testis" was identified and then was removed through a precisely directed incision. Management of the postpubertal undescended testis is controversial. Martin and Menck recommend orchiectomy in patients between puberty and 50 years, whereas Farrer et al. suggest 32 years of age as the ceiling for orchiectomy based on a meta-analysis of the literature.[46, 47] We believe that a clinician who leaves an abdominal testis in a postpubertal male, even one 50 years of age, must assume responsibility for its surveillance. Laparoscopy and open surgery as necessary solves the problem.

A 2-year-old boy with a bilobed scrotal mass on the left and no palpable gonad on the right side underwent inguinal exploration elsewhere. He was found to have crossed testicular ectopia on the side explored. Because of the possibility of occult polyorchidism with crossed testicular ectopia, we performed laparoscopy.[48] The crossing testicular vessels and vas passed over the midline and disappeared into the contralateral inguinal canal; there was no polyorchidism. Laparoscopic findings in crossed testicular ectopia have been described previously.[49]

A muscular 6.5-ft-tall 15-year-old had a large varicocele and mildly diminished testicular size on that side. He also had very significant lower extremity venous varicosities and a right testis that chronically dislocated into his inguinal canal during sports. He wanted the testis anchored, but was not anxious for a contralateral incision for the varicocele, so we attempted pelviscopic clip ligation at the same anesthetic as orchiopexy. We had difficulty getting two Hulka clips to occlude his wide spermatic vessel leash, which was buried deep in retroperitoneal fat. The varicocele recurred; indeed, it probably was not affected by the clip application.

The Future of Genitourinary Celiopelviscopy

Celiopelviscopy has a natural role as the first step in management for boys with nonpalpable testes. The procedure is both diagnostic and therapeutic. We do not believe there is a major indication for other imaging modalities; even if these were completely reliable, they are limited in being able only to either confirm and locate or deny the presence of a gonad. If one accepts the value of prophylactic fixation of a solitary testis, then almost all patients with a nonpalpable testis will require some additional operative step at the time of laparoscopy. With laparoscopic assessment of the supracanalicular testis, the operator can determine the appropriate subsequent operative steps. For an atrophic high testis with a normal contralateral mate, orchiectomy is a likely solution and this can be performed through a small precisely directed incision over the testis, if not through a larger pelviscopic sheath. If testicular salvage is advisable, endoscopic assessment of the spermatic vessels helps distinguish testes amenable to standard orchiopexy from those that will require a Fowler-Stephens procedure. Furthermore, the endoscope adds the option of spermatic vessel clipping for staged Fowler-Stephens orchiopexy. Endoscopic observation of blind-ending vessels is proof of testicular absence and further exploration is not necessary, although contralateral orchiopexy is recommended. Endoscopic observation of normal anatomy at the internal inguinal ring justifies inguinal exploration, but if this reveals no gonad distal to the vessels, testicular absence can be declared without further exploration. Naslund, Gearhart, and Jeffs advocated celiopelviscopy in combination with human chorionic gonadotropin stimulation.[18] Misconstrued monorchia, that is, a missed supracanalicular testis, is a potential time bomb. Brothers et al. reviewed 13 instances of testicular tumors arising in patients ranging from 14 to 49 years of age believed to be missing the testis that later became malignant. Four of these patients had undergone previous explorations, which failed to locate the gonad.[50] For patients with a nonpalpable testis, the mission of the urologist is to locate and treat the gonad or prove its absence. Celiopelviscopy facilitates this goal and permits useful adjunctive measures, such as staging Fowler-Stephens orchiopexy.[51]

Celiopelviscopy has other pediatric surgical and urologic applications. It is of value in the evaluation of children with ambiguous genitalia. Peritoneoscopy has been applied to the diagnosis and treatment of ventriculoperitoneal shunts.[52, 53] Endoscopic application of fibrin glue has been utilized successfully for hepatic trauma.[54] Horsch has used the endoscope to diagnose acute appendicitis.[55] The endoscope can visualize an inguinal hernia easily, which is occasionally a problematic diagnosis that must be resolved by an incision.

A potential interventional use of celiopelviscopy is endoscopic orchiectomy in patients with atrophic testes above the internal ring. We expect that endoscopic clip ligation or suture ligation with extracorporeal and intracorporeal knotting techniques may be helpful for the management of varicocele, although more experience is necessary using Semm's pelviscopic instruments rather than the conventional Hulka clip applicator, with which we failed. Semm's devices probably will find application in traditional urologic endoscopic interventions, such as endopyelotomy. The distal ureter is readily visible through a laparoscope and stone removal or ablation could be mastered through this avenue.[17] Pelviscopic access to obstructed distal ureters also might permit new means of decompression, such as placement of an internal stent between dilated ureter and bladder—going *around* an area of obstruction. Ureteral function might become amenable to measurement via pelviscopic access. Endoscopic ablation of tumors using electrofulguration and lasers is already successful from the inside of the urinary tract, and celiopelviscopy may extend the application of these modalities from the outside as well. Gynecologic experience has validated the role of celiopelviscopy for the diagnosis and treatment of intra-abdominal adhesions, although similar applications in general surgical practice have been slow to take hold. In Kiel, Semm has performed laparoscopic incidental appendectomy in over 150 patients since 1980 without a single complication. Future applications of the laparoscope, which had its origin as a modified cystoscope, will be limited only by imagination. Whatever the future may bring, there is little doubt that celiopelviscopy is a preferable substitute for many laparotomies and a substantial number of abdominal and pelvic interventions.

References

1. Cruise FR: The utility of the endoscope as an aid in the diagnosis and treatment of disease. *Dublin Q J Med Sci* 1865; 39:329–363.
2. Jacobeus HC: Ueber die moglichkeit die zystoskopie bei untersuchung seroser hohlungen anzuwenden. *Munch Med Wochenschr* 1910; 57:2090–2092.
3. Werner R: Sterilisierung der frau durch tubenverkochung. *Chirurgie* 1934; 6:843–845.
4. Bosch PF: Laparoskopie. *Schweiz Z Krankenhaus-u Anstaltsw* 1936; 6:62–70.
5. Palmer R: La celioscopie gynecologique. *Rapport du Prof Mocquot Acad de Chir* 1946; 72:363–368.
6. Semm K: *Operative Manual for Endoscopic Abdominal Surgery.* Chicago, Year Book Medical Publishers, 1987.
7. Cortesi N, Ferrari P, Zambarda E, et al: Diagnosis of bilateral abdominal cryptorchidism by laparoscopy. *Endoscopy* 1976; 8:33–34.
8. Uson AC: Re: Laparoscopy for cryptorchidism. *J Urol* 1982; 128:829–830.
9. Silber SJ, Cohen R: Laparoscopy for cryptorchidism. *J Urol* 1980; 124:928–929.
10. Scott JES: Laparoscopy as an aid in the diagnosis and management of the impalpable testis. *J Pediatr Surg* 1982; 7:14–16.
11. Lowe DH, Brock WA, Kaplan GW: Laparoscopy for localization of nonpalpable testes. *J Urol* 1984; 131:728–729.
12. Malone PS, Guiney EJ: The value of laparoscopy in localising the impalpable undescended testis. *Br J Urol* 1984; 56:429–431.
13. Boddy SM, Corkery JJ, Gornall P: The place of laparoscopy in the management of the impalpable testis. *Br J Surg* 1985; 72:918–920.
14. Manson AL, Terhune D, Jordan G, et al: Preoperative laparoscopic localization of the nonpalpable testis. *J Urol* 1985; 134:919–920.
15. Weiss RM, Seashore JH: Laparoscopy in the management of the nonpalpable testis. *J Urol* 1987; 138:382–385.
16. Bloom DA, Ayers JWT, McGuire EJ: The role of laparoscopy in management of nonpalpable testes. *J d'Urologie* 1988; 94:465–470.
17. Das S, Amar AD: The impact of laparoscopy on modern urologic practice. *Urol Clin North Am* 1988; 15:537–540.
18. Naslund MJ, Gearhart JP, Jeffs RD: Laparoscopy: Its selected use in patients with unilateral nonpalpable testes after human chorionic gonadotropin stimulation. *J Urol* 1989; 142:108–110.
19. Guiney EJ, Corbally M, Malone PS: Laparoscopy and the management of the impalpable testis. *Br J Urol* 1989; 63:313–316.
20. DeCherney A: Complications in laparoscopy, in Weiss RM (ed): *Laparoscopy: Its Role in Management of Nonpalpable Testis. Dialogues in Pediatric Urology.* Pearl River, New York, William J. Miller, 1988, pp 7–8.
21. Rajfer J: *Urologic Endocrinology.* Philadelphia, WB Saunders Co, 1986.

22. Levitt SB, Kogan SJ, Engel RM, et al: The impalpable testis: A rational approach to management. *J Urol* 1978; 120:515–520.
23. Jones PG: Undescended testes. *Aust Paediatr J* 1966; 2:36–48.
24. Scorer CG: The descent of the testis. *Arch Dis Child* 1964; 39:605–609.
25. Betran-Brown F, Villegas-Alvarez F: Clinical classification for undescended testes: Experience in 1,010 orchidopexies. *J Pediatr Surg* 1988; 23:444–447.
26. Jackson MB, Gough MH, Dudley NE: Anatomical findings at orchiopexy. *Br J Urol* 1987; 59:568–571.
27. Krabbe S, Skakkebaek NE, Berthelsen JG, et al: High incidence of undetected neoplasia in maldescended testes. *Lancet* 1979; 1:999–1001.
28. Kogan SJ, Gill B, Bennett B, et al: Human monorchism: A clinicopathological study of unilateral absent testes in 65 boys. *J Urol* 1986; 135:758–761.
29. Ben-Menachem Y, DeBerardinis MC, Salinas R: Localization of intra-abdominal testes by selective testicular arteriography: A case report. *J Urol* 1974; 112:493–494.
30. Greenberg SH, Ring EJ, Pollack HM, et al: The falsely positive gonadal venogram: Presence of a pampiniform plexus without a gonad. *J Urol* 1981; 125:887–888.
31. Wolverson MK, Jagannadharao B, Sundram M, et al: CT in localization of impalpable cryptorchid testes. *Am J Radiol* 1980; 134:725–729.
32. White JJ, Shaker IJ, Oh KS, et al: Herniography: A diagnostic refinement in the management of cryptorchidism. *Am Surg* 1973; 39:624–629.
33. Weiss RM, Carter AR, Rosenfield AT: High resolution real-time ultrasonography in the localization of the undescended testis. *J Urol* 1986; 135:936–938.
34. Kogan BA, Hricak H, Tanagho EA: Magnetic resonance imaging in genital anomalies. *J Urol* 1987; 138:1028–1030.
35. Hinman F Jr: Survey: Localization and operation for nonpalpable testes. *Urology* 1987; 30:193–198.
36. Gearhart JP, Jeffs RD: Diagnostic maneuvers in cryptorchidism. *Semin Urol* 1988; 6:79–83.
37. Steinhardt GF, Kroovand RL, Perlmutter AD: Orchiopexy: Planned 2-stage technique. *J Urol* 1985; 133:534–535.
38. Stephens FD: Fowler-Stephens orchiopexy. *Semin Urol* 1988; 6:103–106.
39. Silber SJ, Kelly J: Successful autotransplantation of an intra-abdominal testis to the scrotum by microvascular technique. *J Urol* 1976; 115:452–454.
40. Duckett JW, personal communication, 1982.
41. Ransley PG, Vordermark JS, Caldamone AA, et al: Preliminary ligation of the gonadal vessels prior to orchiopexy for the intra-abdominal testicle. *World J Urol* 1984; 2:266–268.
42. Pascual JA, Villaneuva-Meyer J, Salido E, et al: Recovery of testicular blood flow following ligation of testicular vessels. *J Urol* 1989; 142:549–552.
43. Oesch I, Ransley PG: Unilaterally impalpable testis. *Eur Urol* 1987; 13:324–326.
44. Harris BH, Webb HW, Wilkinson AH Jr, et al: Protection of the solitary testis. *J Pediatr Surg* 1982; 17:950–952.
45. Bellinger MF, Abramowitz HB, Brantley S, et al: Orchiopexy: An experimental study of the effect of surgical techniques on testicular histology. *J Urol* 1989; 142:553–555.
46. Martin DC, Menck HR: The undescended testis: Management after puberty. *J Urol* 1975; 114:77–79.

47. Farrer JH, Walker H, Rajfer J: Management of the postpubertal cryptorchid testis: A statistical review. *J Urol* 1985; 134:1071–1076.
48. Gandia VM, Arrizabalaga M, Leiva O, et al: Polyorchidism discovered as testicular torsion associated with an undescended atrophic contralateral testis: A surgical solution. *J Urol* 1987; 137:743–744.
49. Gornall PG, Pender DJ: Crossed testicular ectopia detected by laparoscopy. *Br J Urol* 1987; 59:283.
50. Brothers LR III, Weber CH Jr, Ball TP Jr: Anorchism versus cryptorchidism: The importance of a diligent search for intra-abdominal testes. *J Urol* 1978; 119:707–708.
51. Bloom DA: Two-step orchiopexy with pelviscopic clip ligation of the spermatic vessels. *J Urol* 1991, in press.
52. Rogers BM, Vries JK, Talbert JL: Laparoscopy in the diagnosis and treatment of malfunctioning ventriculo-peritoneal shunts in children. *J Pediatr Surg* 1978; 13:247–253.
53. Morgan WW Jr: The use of peritoneoscopy in the diagnosis and treatment of complications of ventriculoperitoneal shunts in children. *J Pediatr Surg* 1979; 4:180–181.
54. Ishitani MB, McGahren ED, Sibley DA, et al: Laparoscopically applied fibrin glue in experimental liver trauma. *J Pediatr Surg* 1989; 24:867–871.
55. Horsch RF: Laparoscopy in the diagnosis of acute appendicitis. *Contemp Surg* 1989; 34:11–16.

Endocrine Abnormalities in Children Associated With Ambiguous Genitalia: Diagnosis and Management

Bruce Blyth, M.D., F.R.A.C.S.

Lecturer in Surgery/Urology, University of Pennsylvania School of Medicine; Attending Urologist, Children's Hospital of Philadelphia, Philadelphia, Pennsylvania

Basic Principles in Sexual Differentiation

General Principles

The phenotypic development of the normal embryo is regulated by the differentiation of the embryonic gonad and the endocrine secretions from this gonad. This fundamental concept was elucidated by Alfred Jost[1] in a series of classic experiments. He established that the development of a female phenotype does not require the presence of a fetal gonad. In contrast, male development proceeds only when a functioning testis is present. In the presence of a testis the paramesonephric (müllerian) ducts disappear, while the mesonephric ducts (wolffian) and urogenital sinus differentiate into the male urogenital tract and external male genitalia. Jost established that the testis exerted these effects by an endocrine mechanism, and was able to deduce that at least two hormones were essential for the development of a male, androgens that produced virilization of the embryo and a second hormone excreted by the fetal testis that induced the regression of the paramesonephric ducts.[2] This is now known as antimüllerian hormone. Jost then formulated the classic dogma that sexual differentiation is a sequential, ordered, and relatively straightforward process (Fig 1).

Basic Factors in Sexual Development

Determination of Chromosomal Sex

Chromosomal sex is determined at fertilization. The fertilizing sperm provides either an X chromosome, resulting in a 46-XX zygote (female geno-

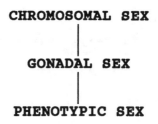

CHROMOSOMAL SEX

|

GONADAL SEX

|

PHENOTYPIC SEX

FIG 1.
Sequence of events in sexual differentiation.

type), or a Y chromosome, resulting in a 46-XY zygote (male genotype). The chromosomal composition can be determined by karyotyping, which is an array of the chromosomes from a single cell in metaphase.[3] The presence of an X chromosome also can be determined at times from a buccal smear,[4] but the usefulness of this is limited in the neonatal assessment of sexual ambiguity, since a Barr body is present in only 20% of infant female cells.

The genetic material necessary for the development of the normal testes is carried on the short arm of the Y chromosome. Genes that are necessary for normal male development also are carried on the X chromosome, and for the full phenotypic development of both males and females, genes from the autosomes are necessary in addition. At least 19 genes are involved in sex determination in humans.[5]

Individuals who have an XXY, XXXY, XXXXY, or XXXX+Y karyotype develop along masculine lines which, although imperfect, are not ambiguous. This clinical observation demonstrates that the presence of the Y chromosome provides the signal for testicular development that is not inhibited by the presence of two or more X chromosomes. Normal testicular development, however, is imperfect, with seminiferous tubular dysgenesis and azoospermia the rule. Other associated anomalies include tall stature, disproportionately long legs, and gynecomastia, with increasing mental retardation as the number of additional X chromosomes increases.

Testis Determining Factor Gene

The testis determining factor (TDF) gene is that segment of DNA that provides the signal for differentiation of the gonad into a testis. This genetic locus has been identified on the distal portion of the short arm of the Y chromosome,[6] and now has been cloned. The TDF gene is localized to within a 160-kilobase segment of DNA.[7] This gene codes for a protein that contains a series of zinc fingers, a motif characteristic of proteins that bind DNA or RNA. Thus, the next step is to find the gene it is regulating, which most likely is present on another chromosome. One very plausible theory of the action of the TDF gene is that it is regulating the rate of growth of the somatic cells in the gonadal ridge. In the presence of the TDF gene, the cells divide more rapidly to form a testis.[8]

In the past, the TDF gene was considered one and the same as the gene coding for the H-Y antigen. The H-Y antigen is a membrane antigen that triggers the rejection of male-to-female grafts in inbred mice.[9] It now has been shown convincingly using cytotoxic T-cell assays that the Tdy (the TDF gene in mice) and H-Y antigen can be separated by mutation in the mouse, and that the TDF and H-Y antigen can be mapped to very different regions of the Y chromosome in the human.[10] The H-Y antigen, however, may prove to play an important role in the maturation of spermatozoa.[11]

Differentiation of the Testis and Ovary

The gonad develops as a thickening, the genital ridge, along the ventral cranial area of the mesonephros and from the migration of the primordial germ cells (Fig 2). The somatic elements of the gonads are derived from mesonephric cells that migrate into the area of the genital ridge very early in development, the mesenchyme, and the coelomic epithelium.[12] The genital ridges initially are devoid of germ cells, which are identified first on the dorsal endoderm of the yolk sac at 24 days of gestation.[13] The primordial germ cells migrate by ameboid action to the gonadal ridge via the mesenchyme of the mesentery (see Fig 2) and appear to be attracted to the gonadal area by a chemotactic factor.[14] Soon after reaching the gonad, the primordial germ cells are enclosed in specific germ-cell compartments where their proliferation and differentiation is regulated by the surrounding somatic cells.

The gonad is indifferent until approximately 45 days' gestation, when in

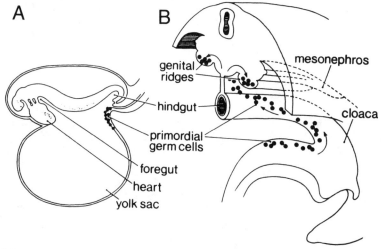

FIG 2.
A, schematic drawing showing the site of origin of the germ cells in the wall of the yolk sac in a 3-week-old embryo. **B,** migratory path of the primordial germ cells along the wall of the yolk sac and dorsal mesentery and into the genital ridge. (From Langman J: *Medical Embryology: Human Development-Normal and Abnormal,* 4th ed. Baltimore, Williams & Wilkins Co, 1986. Used by permission.)

the male the TDF gene triggers differentiation, which is characterized by three consecutive events. Initially, the germ cells and Sertoli cells become enclosed as testicular cords. Next, differentiation of the steroid-producing Leydig cells occurs in the extracordal compartment and, finally, the testis becomes rounded.

Differentiation of the ovary does not occur until significantly later than the testis, around 80 days' gestation. Three events occur in the early stages of ovarian development. The first event observed is the initiation of meiotic prophase. Much later, the diplotene oocyte is enclosed in the germ cell compartment, the follicle. Third, steroid-producing cells in the extrafollicular compartment are differentiated. The production of hormones from the differentiating ovary occurs at the same time as the onset of testosterone synthesis in the male,[15] although the production of estrogens plays no known role in the phenotypic development.

Determination of Phenotypic Sex

The development of phenotypic sex is governed by the endocrine action. When testicular secretions are present, a male phenotype is induced, whereas female differentiation is not dependent on the presence of an ovary and therefore does not require secretions from the embryonic gonad. There are two types of secretions from the fetal testis necessary for male development, a müllerian-inhibiting substance and androgen.

Antimüllerian Hormone.—Antimüllerian hormone, also known as müllerian-inhibiting substance or factor, is a peptide hormone that acts in the male to induce regression of the paramesonephric (müllerian) ducts. It is formed by the embryonic testis soon after the onset of differentiation of the spermatic tubules and is the first secretory function of the testis. The inhibiting substance is a glycoprotein (mol wt 70,000) formed by the spermatogenic tubules.[16, 17] The hormone has been purified,[18] cloned,[19] and its gene mapped to the tip of the short arm of chromosome 19.[20]

Antimüllerian hormone may prove to be a key in the expression of the TDF gene. When added to fetal rat ovaries explanted in organ culture, it induces differentiation of seminiferous cordlike structures.[21] Further, antimüllerian hormone has been shown to inhibit the aromatase activity in fetal rat ovaries, thus dramatically decreasing the conversion of testosterone to estradiol.[22] The release of testosterone that follows when antimüllerian hormone is added to the explants of rat ovarian tissue then induces the formation of the seminiferous cordlike structures. Since normal testicular differentiation can still occur with isolated defects in antimüllerian hormone biosynthesis, it is not the only factor involved in the differentiation of the testis. Antimüllerian hormone can be detected in human testicular tissue up to the age of 6 years and may continue to play a trophic role in the differentiation of the testis beyond its initial formation.[23]

Androgen Secretion.—The second substance secreted by the fetal testis was identified by Jost as an androgen, later deduced to be testosterone.[24] Testosterone formation by the fetal testis commences shortly after the differentiation of the spermatogenic tubules and concomitantly with the histological differentiation of the Leydig cells of the testis.[24] Testosterone acts both within the fetal testis, where it has a role in promoting maturation of the spermatogonia, and beyond the testis, where its paracrine and endocrine actions play an essential role in the development of the male phenotype.

There are at least five separate genetic defects in the human known to cause inadequate testosterone synthesis, with incomplete virilization of the male embryo during embryogenesis,[25] and other defects of steroid synthesis that result in excesses of androgens. Therefore, a knowledge of steroid synthesis is pertinent to the understanding of intersex anomalies. An outline can be seen in Figure 3. While the differentiated testis and ovary possess the enzymatic pathways necessary to produce steroid hormones, the adrenal gland is often responsible for the production of excess androgens and mineralocorticoids in genetic defects of cortisol synthesis (see Fig 3 for

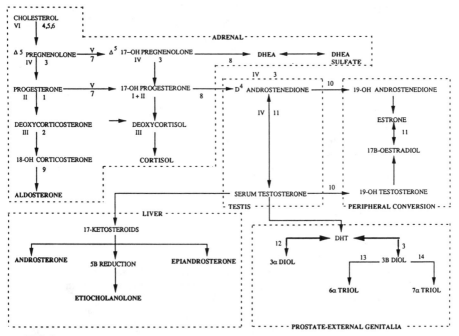

FIG 3.
A diagrammatic representation of the steroid biosynthetic pathways in the adrenal, gonads, liver, and external genitalia. The Roman numerals I to VI correspond to enzymes whose deficiency results in congenital hyperplasia. The numbers 1 through 14 correspond to the different enzymes implicated in the cascade: 1 to 21-hydroxylase; 2 to 11-hydroxylase; 3 to 3-b-hydroxydehydrogenase; 4 to 20α hydroxylase; 5 to 20-22 desmolase; 6 to 22α hydroxylase; 7 to 17α hydroxylase; 8 to 17-20 desmolase; 9 to 18-hydroxylase; 10 to 19-hydroxylase (aromatase); 11 to 17α-ketoreductase; 12 to 3α-hydroxydehydrogenase; 13 to 6α hydroxylase; and 14 to 17α hydroxylase.

specific enzyme defects). With the failure of production of cortisol, the increased secretion of adrenocorticotropic hormone by the pituitary stimulates the adrenal with the overproduction of all precursors in the steroid synthetic pathway.

The response of the urogenital sinus and external genitalia to androgen requires the conversion of testosterone to dihydrotestosterone. Testosterone enters the cell by passive diffusion and in the cytoplasm is converted to dihydrotestosterone by the enzyme 5α-reductase. Testosterone or dihydrotestosterone then is bound to the same high-affinity androgen receptor (R) in the cytosol. This receptor is coded for by one or more X-linked genes.[26] The hormone-receptor complexes move into the nucleus, where they bind to chromatin receptor sites composed of DNA and protein. Transcription RNA polymerase allows the transcription of DNA to messenger RNA, and subsequently new proteins are synthesized. The testosterone-receptor complex is responsible for the regulation of gonadotropin secretion by the hypothalamic-pituitary axis, the regulation of spermatogenesis, and virilization of the mesonephric (wolffian) duct during embryogenesis, whereas the dihydrotestosterone-R complex induces virilization of the urogenital sinus and external genitalia during embryogenesis and is responsible in large part for the maturational events at male puberty.

Three types of single-gene mutations have been identified, each of which affects one step of the pathway; these are the 5α-reductase enzyme, the androgen receptor, and the subsequent phase of hormone action, and each results in hereditary resistance to androgen action and incomplete virilization during embryogenesis, despite the fact that testosterone formation and regression of the müllerian ducts are normal.

Development of the Genital Ducts

The internal genital ducts in both sexes are derived from the mesonephric kidney system. The mesonephric (wolffian) duct drains the mesonephric kidney that develops during the fourth week of gestation and empties into the primitive urogenital sinus. It is from this duct that the ureteric bud arises to induce differentiation of the metanephric kidney. The paramesonephric (müllerian) duct develops at 6 weeks' gestation as an evagination in the coelomic epithelium just lateral to the mesonephros proper, then forms into a tube, the caudal end of which becomes closely attached to the mesonephric duct.[27] Thus, at 7 weeks of intrauterine life the fetus has both mesonephric and paramesonephric primorida, which are capable of forming male and female genital ducts (Fig 4).

At this 7-week stage, the secretion of antimüllerian hormone from the fetal testis promotes the involution of the paramesonephric ducts, while in the absence of this substance the paramesonephric duct persists. In the male, all of the paramesonephric duct reabsorbs except the cranial portion, termed the appendix testis, and the extreme lower end, which contributes to the prostatic utricle.[28] Shortly after the secretion of antimüllerian hormone, the testis also secretes testosterone, which acts to stabilize the mesonephric duct. Both of these hormone actions of the fetal testis occur

INDIFFERENT STAGE

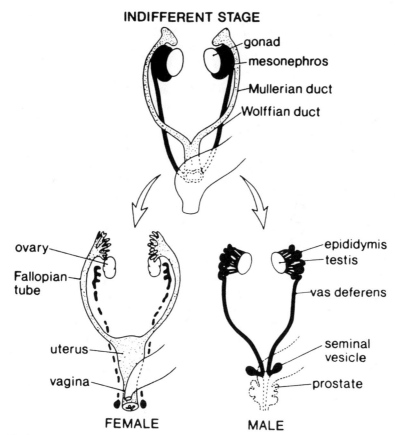

gonad
mesonephros
Mullerian duct
Wolffian duct

ovary
Fallopian tube
uterus
vagina

epididymis
testis
vas deferens
seminal vesicle
prostate

FEMALE   MALE

FIG 4.
Contribution of the wolffian and müllerian ducts and the urogenital tract. (From George FW, Wilson JD: *Campbell's Urology,* 5th ed. Philadelphia, WB Saunders Co, 1986. Used by permission.)

through a paracrine mechanism, i.e., the steroids move from their site of action to the target tissue by local diffusion through the extracellular space. Therefore, the response of the mesonephric and paramesonephric ducts depends on the function of the ipsilateral testis.

Under the influence of testosterone, the mesonephric duct differentiates into the epididymis, the vas deferens, the ejaculatory ducts, and the seminal vesicles (see Fig 4). In the absence of the influence of testosterone, the mesonephric duct involutes and the paramesonephric duct develops into the oviduct, uterus, cervix, and upper vagina.[29]

Development of the Urogenital Sinus and External Genitalia

The development of the external genitalia and the urogenital sinus occurs following division of the cloaca and the formation of the tail fold in the embryo. In the third week of development, a pair of slightly elevated folds (the cloacal folds) unite to form the genital tubercle, which later elongates as a phallus. The portion of the primitive urogenital sinus caudal to the mesonephric ducts forms the definitive urogenital sinus.[30] The segment of the sinus near the bladder is narrow (pelvic urethra), while the segment near the urogenital membrane is expanded (phallic urethra). In the male, under the influence of dihydrotestosterone, the phallic segment of the urogenital sinus then develops into the bulbar and penile urethra. This occurs at 60 to 70 days' gestation, while in the female, development does not occur until much later, nearer 140 days' gestation. In the presence of dihydrotestosterone, the pelvic urethra forms the neck of the primitive bladder and prostatic urethra as far as the utricle, where the müllerian tubercle becomes the seminal colliculus. The glandular part of the prostate develops from endodermal buds from the pelvic urethra.[31] Beyond the prostatic utricle, the pelvic part of the urogenital sinus forms the rest of the prostatic urethra and the membranous urethra.

As the genital folds close over the phallic portion of the sinus and the urethral groove, from proximal to distal, the opening of the urogenital sinus migrates forward along the ventral aspect of the phallus. The genital swellings also meet and fuse to form the scrotum. Meanwhile, under the influence of dihydrotestosterone, the genital tubercle has elongated cylindrically to become the penis. The endodermal edges of the urethral groove fuse to tubularize the penile urethra, while ectoderm has grown in from the glans as a plug that meets the penile urethra and later cavitates as the glanular urethra. When formation of the male urethra is complete at 80 days, the size of the male phallus is not substantially different from that of the female, but under the continued influence of androgens, the external male genitalia grows progressively during pregnancy and at term is much larger than the female phallus. In the absence of dihydrotestosterone, the vesicourethral canal elongates to form the majority of the urethra, while the pelvic part of the urogenital sinus develops into the distal portion of the urethra and the vagina. The vagina begins development with the formation of a solid mass of cells (the uterovaginal plate) between the caudal buds of the paramesonephric ducts and the posterior wall of the urogenital sinus. The cells of the vaginal plate proliferate until around 80 days' gestation, then the plate becomes canalized by the extension of the uterovaginal canal from above and the formation of a lumen from below. By 20 weeks' gestation, the vagina is completely canalized but remains separated from the urogenital sinus by a thin membrane of mesenchymal tissue, the hymen. In the female, the presence of androgenic stimuli after formation of the vaginal opening will not result in posterior fusion of the genital swellings, but only in hypertrophy of the clitoris. The urethral folds do not fuse but form the labia minora, while the genital swellings enlarge to form the labia majora.

Development of Secondary Sex Characteristics

The appearance of secondary sex characteristics at puberty is entirely under the control of the endocrine system. In chronological order, the female development is pubarche (the development of pubic and axillary hair), thelarche (breast enlargement and redistribution of fat), and finally menarche (menses). Pubarche is secondary to an increase in the adrenal production of dehydroepiandrosterone-s (see Fig 3), which stimulates the pilosebaceous apparatus. Ovarian secretion of estrogen under the influence of luteinizing hormone from the pituitary stimulates breast development and the redistribution of fat. The menarche is controlled also by ovarian secretion under the cyclic influence of luteinizing hormone and follicle-stimulating hormone.

In the male, secondary sex characteristics include the appearance of pubic and axillary hair; deepening of the voice; the development of facial hair; and an increase in muscle mass, testicular size, and penile length. Testosterone and dihydrotestosterone effect on all these changes except the pubarche, which is under the influence of dehydroepiandrosterone-S from the adrenal.

Clinical Approach to Problems of Sexual Differentiation

Classification

In order to make a diagnosis in a neonate with a sexual ambiguity, it is necessary to unravel the developmental process that led to the presenting phenotype. The child presents at birth with a summary of its sexual development, while the defect can occur at any step in the path of differentiation. All cases of ambiguous genitalia arise from aberrations in endocrine secretion. Thus, a classification could be organized according to the defect in hormone synthesis or the lack of response by the target organ. It also would have to include an appropriate response to an inappropriate hormone, as occurs with congenital adrenal hyperplasia. However, it is not possible to place in this endocrinological type of classification those cases of ambiguous genitalia in which uncertainty remains about the etiology, such as true hermaphroditism. Therefore, this review will present the most widely accepted classification currently in use, which is based upon the histology of the gonad present, with subclassification according to the etiology, as proposed by Allen.[32] By this gonadal classification, there are five major categories, as follows:

I. Ovary only: female pseudohermaphrodite.
II. Testis only: male pseudohermaphrodite.
III. Ovary plus testis: true hermaphrodite.
IV. Testis plus streak: mixed gonadal dysgenesis.
V. Streak plus streak: pure gonadal dysgenesis.

Hypospadias, micropenis, and cryptorchidism are the results of deficiencies of hormonal secretion in the late embryonic and fetal stages of development, but are not considered in this discussion.

Clinical Presentation

Female Pseudohermaphrodites

This is the most important group, since they constitute 60% to 70% of all intersex cases presenting in the neonatal period. All patients have a 46-XX karyotype; are chromatin-positive, H-Y antigen–and TDF gene–negative; and have exclusively ovarian tissue. The müllerian system develops into fallopian tubes, uterus, and upper vagina, and the wolffian system regresses. Clinically, the virilization of their external genitalia varies from minimal phallic enlargement to almost complete masculinization. As a result of the increase in adrenocorticotropic hormone drive, they also have hyperpigmented skin over their external genitalia and nipples. Female pseudohermaphrodites can be divided in two groups: those fetuses in whom the abnormal masculinization occurs from the presence of inappropriate androgen and those affected by a nonsteroidal mechanism.

Nonsteroidal female pseudohermaphrodites are always associated with significant cloacal or urogenital sinus problems. In a patient with a 46-XX karyotype, the presence of two ovaries and associated urogenital or cloacal abnormalities is diagnostic of these rare problems.

Cases resulting from abnormal androgens constitute the vast majority of female pseudohermaphrodites. The masculinization is limited to the external genitalia and clitoral hypertrophy if the androgenic stimulus is received after 12 weeks' gestation. If the stimulus is received earlier, clitoral hypertrophy still occurs, plus retention of the urogenital sinus and labioscrotal fusion. These patients must be diagnosed correctly, as they should be raised as females. Their prognosis when raised as females is excellent for pubertal development, the attainment of normal female characteristics, sexual activity, and reproduction.

Abnormal androgen may be the result of fetal biosynthetic anomalies (vast majority) or from the maternal source of androgens (either endogenous or exogenous). Fortunately, these cases of maternal androgen origin are now very rare.

Congenital adrenal hyperplasia makes up the vast majority of these cases of female pseudohermaphrodites.[33] There are six types of adrenogenital syndromes, all of which have a defect in the production of cortisol, with secondary increases in the secretion of adrenocorticotropic hormone, and consequent hyperplasia of the adrenals.[34] Only types I through IV are virilizing and cause female pseudohermaphroditism (see Fig 3).

In the type I abnormality, the defect of C21-hydroxylation is localized in the zona fasciculata, but not in the zona granulosa. This results in increased production of 17-hydroxyprogesterone and blocked cortisol production. The concentration of 17-hydroxyprogesterone is of great clinical importance in making the diagnosis. The overproduction of androgens resulting from the block causes the inappropriate masculinizing effect on the urogenital sinus and external genitalia. Cortisol deficiency and the resulting continued adrenocorticotropic hormone stimulation with secondary hyperpigmentation are important other downstream effects of the defect in C21-hydroxylation.

In type II congenital adrenal hyperplasia, the 21-hydroxylase deficiency involves the zona granulosa as well. Thus, in addition to the changes described above, there is also a deficiency of biologically active mineralocorticoid (see Figure 3). The latter results in electrolyte imbalance with salt and water loss, usually requiring treatment.

In type III congenital adrenal hyperplasia, the enzymatic block occurs at the 11-hydroxylase level (see Fig 3). Again, two important proximal metabolites, the 17-hydroxyprogesterone and the androgen, accumulate. Cortisol deficiency and adrenocorticotropic hormone excess are features, but there is also an accumulation of a biologically active and very potent mineralocorticoid, deoxycorticosterone. In the affected children, the electrolyte imbalance with hypokalemic acidosis, hypervolemia, and secondary hypertension can be life-threatening if left untreated.

Type IV congenital adrenal hyperplasia is the only form caused by an enzyme deficiency that results in ambiguity in both male and female. The enzymatic block occurs more proximally at the 3b-ol dehydrogenase level (see Fig 3). It is the rarest of the four forms of congenital adrenal hyperplasia and, as it is associated with the greatest degree of salt wasting, survival is rare. The principal androgen that accumulates proximal to the block is dehydroepiandrosterone, a weak androgen, and thus the degree of virilization encountered in affected females is usually not as severe as that seen in other types of this disorder. Most patients have separate urethral and vaginal orifices. The hormonal deficiencies found are in cortisol and mineralocorticoids, with excess adrenocorticotropic hormone and severe hyponatremia.

All patients with types I through IV congenital adrenal hyperplasia require cortisol replacement. Hydrocortisone sodium succinate 50 mg/m^2 should be given as a bolus, and another 50 to 100 mg/m^2 should be added to the infusion of parenteral fluid over the next 24 hours.[34] Regular monitoring of serum electrolytes and blood pressure measurements are essential to avoid the potential catastrophe of shock or hypokalemic acidosis and hypertension that may occur in most children with female pseudohermaphroditism and mineralocorticoid deficiency or excess, respectively. If profound hypotension and hyperkalemia are present, deoxycorticosterone acetate 1 to 2 mg should be given intramuscularly over 12 to 14 hours. If the patient is in shock, 20 mL/kg of saline must be given in the first hours of therapy.

Male Pseudohermaphrodites

The male pseudohermaphrodites constitute by far the most confusing group in the classification of intersex. In the neonatal period, they present with ambiguity; have a 46-XY karyotype; and are chromatin-negative and H-Y antigen– and TDF gene–positive. They also have exclusively testicular tissue and develop their wolffian system while the müllerian system regresses. In this category, many also present later in life with failure of pubertal development or procreative function. The mechanisms underlying the failure of testosterone synthesis by the testis or the failure of target tissues to respond to circulating testosterone are shown in Figure 5. The secretion of testosterone by the fetal testes is influenced by the gonadotropins, with hypotrophic hypogonadism occurring where there is a deficiency of luteinizing hormone or human chorionic gonadotropin.

Deficient Testosterone Biosynthesis.—Defects in three enzymes involved in the synthesis of steroid hormones have been identified that result in male pseudohermaphroditism and ambiguous genitalia in the neonate. These enzymes are 20-22 desmolase, 3b-ol dehydrogenase, and 17-20 demolase. All three interfere in the cascade production of testosterone and/or cortisol (see Fig 3). The deficiency in 20-22 desmolase or 3b-ol hydrogenase results in death in the majority of affected males. They present with ambiguous external genitalia varying from mild hypospadias to complete failure of masculinization with the presence of a vagina. Most exhibit some element of hypospadias and scrotal fusion. The wolffian ducts are normally developed. They also have darkly pigmented skin and severe salt wasting. A few patients with the 3b-ol dehydrogenase deficiency have survived into adulthood and have shown a mixture of partial virilization and gynecomastia at puberty, but no fertility has been reported.[35] The virilization phenomena are caused by the accumulation of a weak androgen (dehydroepiandrosterone) behind the enzyme block.

A 17-20 desmolase deficiency produces ambiguity with some virilization at the time of puberty. There is no interference with the synthesis of cortisol, no increase in the adrenocorticotropic hormone drive, and no elevation of precursor steroids behind the block,[35] and thus no congenital adrenal hyperplasia. Fertility has not been described so far in the few cases reported in the literature.[35, 36] This syndrome also has been described in one 46-XX female with sexual infantilism.[37]

A deficiency in two further enzymes in the synthesis of steroid hormones, 17α-hydroxylase and 17-keto-reductase, results in the failure of testosterone synthesis. These enzyme deficiencies do not cause ambiguity in the neonatal period and individuals present later in life as amenorrheic phenotypic females. They have a 46-XY karyotype and are chromatin-negative and TDF gene–positive. In the gonads, exclusively testicular tissue is found, with development of the wolffian ducts and regression of the müllerian ducts.

In the 17α-hydroxylase deficiency, the patient presents clinically as a phenotypic female with hypogonadism and the absence of all secondary sex characteristics. Hypertension and hypokalemia alkalosis also are present secondary to the accumulation of deoxycorticosterone behind the block (see Figure 3). There is also an excess of adrenocorticotropic hormone secondary to a virtually undetectable cortisol level (see Fig 3). The aldosterone level is also presumably low, secondary to the high plasma deoxycorticosterone level and depressed angiotensin levels. At puberty they remain infantile female, although some affected individuals with presumed partial deficiency might develop pathologic gynecomastia. Those

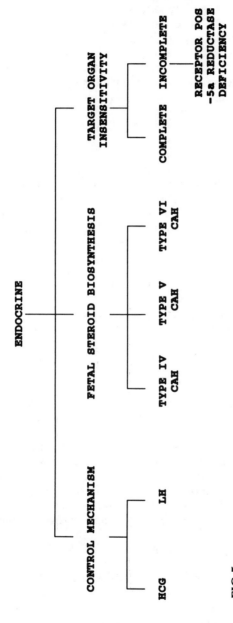

FIG 5.
Schematic representation of different mechanisms implicated in the etiology of male pseudohermaphroditism. *HCG* = human chorionic gonadotropin; *LH* = luteinizing hormone; *CAH* = congenital adrenal hyperplasia.

individuals with partial deficiency also might present at birth with some ambiguity, consisting of varying degrees of hypospadias. This deficiency has been described also in 46-XX subjects who present at puberty with sexual infantilism, amenorrhea, and hypertension.

Males suffering from 17-keto-reductase deficiency have a female phenotype with a blind-ending vagina, but the absence of all müllerian derivatives. They usually have bilaterally undescended testes. There is no defect of secretion of cortisol; thus, there is no excess adrenocorticotropic hormone production and no congenital adrenal hyperplasia (see Fig 3). At puberty, however, because of the increase in luteinizing hormone secretion and some escape through the block, a combination of both virilization and feminization results in phallic enlargement, pubarche, and a variable degree of breast development.

Androgen Insensitivity Syndromes.—The inability of a target organ to respond to circulating testosterone is the result of androgen insensitivity, which can be complete or partial. Complete androgen insensitivity syndromes are rare, occurring in 1 in 20,000 to 1 in 64,000 male births. The incomplete forms are even rarer, with an incidence one-tenth that of the complete form. Unlike the complete forms of androgen insensitivity, the incomplete forms result in ambiguity in the neonatal period. The deficiency is caused by the lack of response of the target organ to the normally secreted androgen. The defect is thought to be localized at the level of the cytoplasmic androgen receptor of the 5α-reductase enzyme, or also to occur with a specific deficiency in this enzyme.

Two major types of defects of the androgen receptor have been described: a quantitative receptor defect (receptor-negative, or AR−) and a qualitative receptor defect (receptor-positive, or AR+). The AR− syndrome implies that the specific intracellular androgen receptors are undetectable (AR−) in all target organs, whereas normal levels of androgen receptors are measured in the AR+ variant. The latter is thought to represent a qualitative defect in the response of the receptor secondary to a structural abnormality therein.[38] These measurements usually are done by fibroblast culture.

Clinically, AR− usually represents the complete androgen insensitivity syndrome, although some cases have been reported with AR+.[38] AR+ is probably responsible for the clinically incomplete form with the 5α-reductase deficiency. This pathophysiologic distinction is probably responsible for the different type of presentation encountered with these syndromes.

Indeed, individuals affected by the complete androgen insensitivity syndrome do not present in the neonatal period with ambiguous genitalia, but rather later in life as phenotypically normal females, best known as suffering from the testicular feminization syndrome. The complete androgen insensitivity syndrome now has been identified as an X-linked mutation that precludes the normal synthesis of the androgen receptor located in the cytosol.[39] These individuals are phenotypically normal, tall, and hairless females with nonambiguous feminine external genitalia and symmetrically undescended gonads. They usually have a shallow vaginal cavity probably corresponding to a vast prostatic utricle. At the time of puberty, normal breasts develop with absent or scanty axillary and pubic hair. There is slight vulval hair development and amenorrhea is the rule. Clinically, they present usually in the postpubertal period for evaluation of primary amenorrhea or less often during the prepubertal period because of inguinal hernias. All of these patients have a 46-XY karyotype, are chromatin-negative, H-Y antigen– and TDF gene–positive, and have exclusively testicular tissue (seminiferous tubules with no spermatogenesis and increased numbers of Leydig cells). The internal ducts develop normally as wolffian ducts and there is regression of all müllerian structures.

The gonads in these patients are at higher risk for malignancy because of the cryptorchidism in this condition, and gonadectomy is recommended. The timing of gonadectomy can be individualized. Since the testis tumors that can occur rarely develop before puberty, surgical intervention is indicated in the prepubertal period only if the presence of the testis in the labia majora or inguinal region results in discomfort or hernia formation. Estrogen therapy will be necessary for individuals who undergo pubertal gonadectomy to ensure normal growth and breast development. When castration is performed postpubertally, estrogen withdrawal symptoms are the rule and estrogen supplements are necessary.

In contrast to the complete androgen insensitivity syndrome, incomplete androgen insensitivity syndromes including AR+ and 5α-reductase deficiency cause ambiguity in the neonatal period. Although the incidence is about one tenth that of the complete form (AR−), innumerable incomplete androgen insensitivity (AR+) phenotypes have been outlined in the literature and their exhaustive description is beyond the scope of this chapter. The important and common characteristics are that the individuals have a 46-XY karyotype and are chromatin-negative and TDF gene–positive. They have exclusively testicular tissue, the internal ducts develop normally and sometimes incompletely (hypoplastic or absent vas) as wolffian ducts, and there is regression of the müllerian structures. There is a minor defect of virilization of the external genitalia, consisting of partial fusion of the labioscrotal folds and some degree of clitoromegaly present at birth, which presents the ambiguity. The gonads are usually symmetrically undescended and there is a short, blind-ending vagina. At puberty, both some virilization and some feminization occurs, including the development of normal pubic hair and gynecomastia. Sex assignment should be individualized and made thoughtfully. The same considerations apply as in the true hermaphrodites and mixed gonadal dysgenesis. The potential for fertility is usually considered nonexistent. Since some virilization is expected at the time of puberty in those assigned the female sex, gonadectomy should be performed during the prepubertal period.

The deficiency in 5α-reductase is a rare syndrome originally described in humans in 1974.[40] The deficit is found in the genital sinus and hepatic tissues. A number of cases have been reported in the Dominican Republic, where a recessive trait seems to be the inheritance pattern.

At puberty in the different forms of androgen insensitivity, despite very low affinity of the cytoplasmic receptors for testosterone, some virilization occurs, because testosterone is secreted in such excess: the voice deepens, the muscle mass increases, and the phallus lengthens. In 5α-reductase–deficient subjects, basal plasma testosterone levels are normal or elevated and plasma dihydrotestosterone levels are normal or decreased. The diagnosis of 5α-reductase deficiency in adults is made by measuring the ratio of testosterone to dihydrotestosterone, which is increased. However, in affected children past infancy, the basal plasma testosterone and dihydrotestosterone are too low for accurate determination of their ratio. This measurement can be done after human chorionic gonadotropin stimulation of the Leydig cells. Imperato-McGinley et al.[41] described a new method of diagnosing this deficiency by measuring the ratio of other C19 and C21 steroids and their 5α-reduced urinary metabolites. Of course, demonstrating that the genital skin is unable to convert testosterone to dihydrotestosterone in tissue culture is the ultimate test for diagnosis.[42]

Although hypospadias with or without undescended testis usually is not considered as an example of intersexuality, it is obviously closely related. With the progress in understanding the different androgen insensitivity syndromes,[38, 41, 43] it is reasonable to postulate that if a very isolated resistance to androgen occurs at a critical time during sexual differentiation, it could lead to incomplete virilization phenomena such as hypospadias.

Klinefelter's Syndrome.—This disorder was described in 1942 by Klinefelter, Reinstein, and Albright.[44] The original description was of a man with bilaterally small and firm testes, varying degrees of impaired sexual maturation, azoospermia, gynecomastia, and elevated levels of urinary gonadotropins. Clearly, these patients are not ambiguous at birth, but imperfect.

The karyotype for this syndrome can be 47-XXY, 46-XX/47-XXY, or even 48-XXXY to 49-XXXXY. The chromatin is positive as well as the H-Y antigen. Such patients have symmetrically descended testes which have normal histology at birth, but show a drastic loss of germ cells in early infancy, followed by progressive tubular hyalinization during adolescence.

These patients usually seek medical attention at puberty because of sexual infantilism, or later in life for infertility, which occurs secondary to primary hypogonadism. The syndrome includes a constellation of physical, biochemical, and hormonal abnormalities. The reader is referred to Leonard et al.[45] for further details.

Hernia Uteri Inguinale.—The persistent müllerian duct syndrome of hernia uteri inguinale is a rare condition resulting from the failure of paracrine secretion of antimüllerian hormone by the Sertoli cells or failure of the müllerian ducts to respond to its secretion. Now that antimüllerian hormone has been purified and immunohistochemical techniques are available to stain for it, testicular biopsies from these patients can be examined to clarify whether it is present. In six patients with this syndrome, antimüllerian hormone was expressed normally in the testicular tissue of two of them. In the other four patients, there was no detectable bioactive or immunoreactive hormone, yet they expressed antimüllerian hormone messenger RNA with a normal transcription initiation site and in the amount expected for their age.[46] This confirms the heterogeneity of the hernia uteri inguinale and suggests that peripheral insensitivity to antimüllerian hormone can be present.

Males affected are not ambiguous at birth and generally present later with symmetrically or asymmetrically undescended testes for orchiopexy or repair of inguinal hernias. The gonadal tissue is exclusively testicular, but both wolffian and müllerian duct derivatives are present with a vas and epididymis alongside an ipsilateral uterus, fallopian tube, and upper vagina. The external genitalia are nonambiguous male with unilateral or bilateral cryptorchidism. Rare cases of associated hypospadias have been reported.

XX Male Reversal.—The incidence of XX male reversal is approximately 1 in 20,000 to 1 in 24,000 male births, making it a rare disorder. The affected individuals are not ambiguous at birth and have a normal male phenotype. They have a 46-XX karyotype, are chromatin-positive, and also may be H-Y antigen–positive. This group of patients has been the key in isolating the gene controlling the formation of the testis. By restriction enzyme fragmentation of the X chromosomes and the use of DNA probes, it has been shown that the majority of the XX sex-reversed males contain fragments of DNA from the short arm of the Y chromosome in the distal end of the short arm of the X chromosome.[47–49] These patients have exclusively testicular tissue and develop the wolffian system while the müllerian ducts regress.

The external genitalia are nonambiguous male phenotype, very similar to Klinefelter's syndrome, but with a more frequent association with hypospadias and an average height less than normal. The testes are small and firm but bilaterally descended. The penile length is normal or slightly shorter than normal, and they also develop gynecomastia and hyalinization of the seminiferous tubules at puberty with incomplete pubarche. Infertility occurs secondary to hypogonadism.

True Hermaphrodites

At birth, true hermaphrodites present with ambiguous genitalia and asymmetry of their gonads. They constitute 10% of the intersex pool.[35] A 46-XX karyotype is found in 57% (57% to 80%) of these patients.[50] The others have a 46-XY pattern[51] (13%) or a mosaic with 46XX/XY (31%). The chromatin is positive in 70%, but the H-Y antigen is also positive in the majority of these individuals. This is thought to represent a translocation of the testis derminants from the Y chromosome to the X chromosome in patients with 46-XX karyotype.

True hermaphrodites have ovarian and testicular tissue present in the same individual. This may take the form of an ovary on one side and a testis on the other, or both components in the same gonad representing an ovotestis. Internal duct differentiation follows the appropriate ipsilateral gonad. When an ovotestis is present, the differentiation of the ducts is variable. A uterus is almost always present[42] and may be hypoplastic or unicornous.[35]

Although the appearance of the external genitalia may span the spectrum from feminine with slight clitoral prominence to full masculinization, a tendency to maleness with asymmetrically descended gonads and hypospadias predominates in 75% of patients.[42] The changes at puberty are variable, but generally correlate with the gonadal tissue present. Sex assignment should be made thoughtfully. The presence or absence of an adequate phallus both functionally and cosmetically is a cornerstone in the decision process.

Three cases of true hermaphroditism and pregnancy have been reported in the literature.[52–54] These three cases constitute the only indication that there might be potential for fertility in true hermaphrodites. In at least two of the three individuals, the karyotype was 46-XX. There is also a report of spermatogenesis in the testis of true hermaphrodites.[55] All these observations are indicative of the possible fertility potential in true hermaphrodites, but further studies are required.

Mixed Gonadal Dysgenesis

In this group with sexual ambiguity, the gonads are classically asymmetrical. Most of these patients have a mosaic 46-XY/45-XO karyotype. Their gonadal composition is characterized by testicular tissue on one side and a dysgenetic gonad (streak) on the other. The testis is composed of Sertoli cells and Leydig cells, but no germinal cells are present. The streak gonad appears similar to the ovarian stroma, but without oocytes. It occurs most probably secondary to paracrine insufficiency from the testis; the müllerian duct usually persists unilaterally or bilaterally. The testis is often provided with a fallopian tube rather than a vas and an epididymis. The streak gonad is usually drained by a müllerian duct. A bicornuate or unicornous uterus is generally present.

Malignancy will develop in about 15% to 25% of the streak gonads, usually in the form of gonadoblastomas and/or dysgerminomas.[42] Individuals with a 46-XY karyotype are at a much higher risk than are those with a mosaic pattern. Individuals tend to virilize and have gynecomastia at the time of puberty. No fertility has been reported so far, thus sex assignment should be individualized. The response of the phallus to androgenic stimulation should be assessed in borderline cases, but the female gender is usually preferred for the following reasons:

1. The development of the phallus is usually inadequate for functional and cosmetic surgical results.
2. The presence of a mosaic pattern with 46-XY/45-XO predisposes them to short stature.
3. These individuals are infertile, and a bilateral gonadectomy is essential in view of the high malignancy potential of those gonads, particularly those with Y cell–bearing lines.

Patients assigned as female require gonadectomy, clitoroplasty, and vaginoplasty. Those assigned to the male gender usually should undergo removal of any dysgenetic gonadal tissue and repair of the usually severe hypospadias.

Pure Gonadal Dysgenesis

With pure gonadal dysgenesis, there is no ambiguity in the neonatal period but patients usually present later in life as phenotypic females with sexual infantilism. They have variable karyotype (45-XO, 46-XX, 46-XY) and corresponding chromatin and TDF gene. There are bilateral streak gonads, symmetrically undescended and developed, yet the müllerian derivatives are hypoplastic and the wolffian system has regressed. Beyond these similarities, the clinical picture of these patients is variable, depending primarily upon their chromosomal configuration. Subjects with a 45-XO karyotype, for example, exhibit all the stigmata of Turner's syndrome, with short stature, webbed neck, shieldlike chest, and other characteristics. Individuals with a 46-XX karyotype are usually normal in height, even tall, but present at puberty with sexual infantilism and amenorrhea. Patients with a 46-XY karyotype have similar complaints and appearance, but their streak gonads have a high malignancy potential. Dysgerminoma and/or gonadoblastoma are particularly frequent and present clinically with pelvic mass and/or signs of virilization. Thus, bilateral gonadectomy is essential at the time of diagnosis for patients with a 46-XY karyotype.

Diagnosis

The first observation of ambiguous genitalia is made immediately at the time of delivery and the uncertainty that ensues directs the delivery room physicians to seek rapid assistance with two specific goals: (1) accurate sex assignment, and (2) detection of specific underlying endocrinopathies (particularly of the salt-losing variety) that may endanger the infant. The algorithm for the diagnosis of intersex proposed in Figures 6 and 7 allows the clinician to identify newborns with potential electrolyte imbalance rapidly and gives a working diagnosis that will be accurate in 90% of cases.

The maternal history of androgen exposure, either endogenous or exogenous, is usually very easy to obtain. As well, a family history of neonatal death is a clue for a diagnosis of congenital adrenal hyperplasia, although this still may be present in an infant with either male or female pseudohermaphroditism. The physical examination in that case will orient the diagnosis according to whether or not the gonads are symmetrically or asymmetrically descended. Although ovotestes have been reported to descend completely into the bottom of the labioscrotal folds, generally only testicular material fully descends. If there are palpable inguinal gonads, the diagnoses of gonadal female, Turner's syndrome, and pure gonadal dysgenesis can be eliminated. Even in what appears to be a fully virilized infant, the presence of impalpable gonads should raise the possibility of a severely virilized female pseudohermaphrodite with congenital adrenal hyperplasia. If

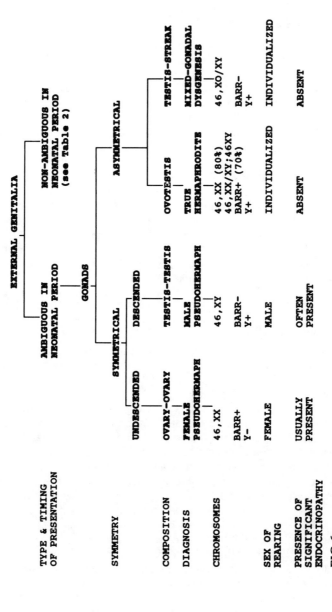

FIG 6.
Diagnostic algorithm for infant presenting with ambiguous genitalia. (From Blyth, Churchill, Houle, et al: Intersex, in Gillenwater JY, Grayhack JT, Howards SS, et al (eds): *Adult and Pediatric Urology*, vol 2, 2nd ed. Chicago, Mosby–Year Book, Inc., 1991, pp 2141–2171.

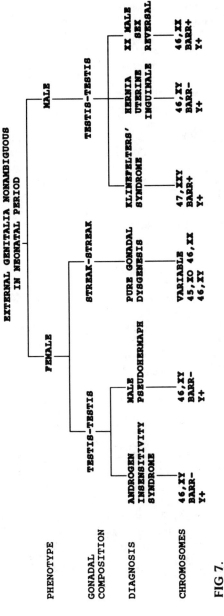

FIG 7.
Diagnostic algorithm of intersex present in the non-neonatal period. The 46,XX Barr + Y + karotype is as detected by the techniques of restriction fragment length polymorphism.

the scrotum or labioscrotal folds are rugated with increased pigmentation, the possibility of increased adrenocorticotropic hormone as part of the adrenogenital syndrome is suggested. The measurement of phallic length and comparison with known nomograms[56] is important, especially in consideration for penile reconstruction. A rectal examination, ultrasound, or retrograde genitogram may detect the servix and uterus, confirming müllerian duct structures. This rules out male pseudohermaphrodites, except those with hernia uteri inguinalis and those with dysgenetic gonads. While the physical examination has its rewards at the extreme ends of the spectrum, it has its limitations in the majority of cases. The establishment of chromosomal sex and measurements of different key biochemical metabolites, therefore, remains essential.

The chromosomal sex is best determined by karyotyping, which can be done within 48 hours with activated T lymphocytes; however, the regular 72-hour lymphocyte culture is preferable. A reliable result can be achieved by microscopy without photography and banding at 3 to 4 days. A complete karyotype with banding and photography can be achieved in 6 to 7 days. The buccal smear is inadequate for definitive sex assignment, but is a useful tool.[57] The same buccal smear can be stained with quinacrine dyes and examined by fluorescent microscopy to define the distal end of the long arm of the Y chromosome.

The determination of a raised plasma 17-OH progesterone level is diagnostic of congenital adrenal hyperplasia. This measurement should be done after 48 hours of life, as earlier levels can reflect the presence of maternal progesterone. The clinical presence of hypokalemic alkalosis or hypertension may reflect underlying deficiencies of cortisol and mineralocorticoids or an excess of deoxycorticosterone, and require urgent correction. Once the diagnosis of congenital adrenal hyperplasia is made from the elevated levels of 17-OH progesterone, further biochemical measurements of the various precursors can identify the exact enzymatic block. Further evaluations are strongly recommended to determine the status of the urogenital sinus, the ductal system, and gonads by radiology, endoscopy, ultrasonography, laparotomy, and gonadal biopsy.[57] Only female pseudohermaphrodites and those with Turner's syndrome (46-XO) do not require gonadal biopsy. All other infants presenting in the neonatal period with ambiguous genitalia should have a biopsy. In the future, the wider dissemination of steroid immunoassays may permit gonadal males with blocks of testosterone production and resultant genital ambiguity to be diagnosed precisely biochemically, as may assays to measure deficiencies of 5α-reductase or androgen binding, without the need for gonadal biopsy.

Once all the above relevant information had been obtained, the sex assignment should be made thoughtfully with the considerations outlined following paramount in the decision.

Phallic Size

A comparison of the stretched penile length and corporal body girth with known growth curves must be obtained.[56, 58] The growth response to androgen stimulus can be a key factor in distinguishing borderline cases. Currently, despite a much deeper understanding of the development of sexual identity, phallic size is still believed to be the most significant criterion in gender assignment in the newborn.[56, 59] Although nomograms are available for penile length (see earlier), the minimum size of phallus required to avoid male inadequacy is not clearly defined.[56] At this institution, we recommend gender conversion when the stretched length of the neonatal phallus is less than 1 cm.

Fertility Potential and Risk of Gonadal Malignancy

Except for female pseudohermaphrodites and rare cases of true hermaphrodites, fertility potential usually is considered nonexistent in mixed gonadal dysgenesis, and is uncertain in male pseudohermaphroditism. On the other hand, more than 50% of true hermaphrodites will have menses at the time of puberty.[55] The necessity of gonadectomy for dysgenetic testes must be weighed against the fertility potential in those with Y cell–bearing lines in deciding on sex assignment. Gonadoblastomas are tumors composed of three elements: large germ cells, sex cord derivatives, and stromal elements. Even though gonadoblastomas are not malignant, these tumors frequently contain dysgerminoma elements that can metastasize. The risk of neoplasia in streak gonads with an XY karyotype, as mentioned earlier, is much larger than in streak gonads with XX chromosomes. Cryptorchid testes, even when not associated with intersex, also have an increased risk of malignancy.

Patient or Family Wishes

Family history, culture, and preferences, particularly if based on prior experience, are of major importance. Parental wishes may be very dominant or predetermined in dictating one sex of rearing over another. This is most often based on longstanding cultural bias and may not be alterable by any medical advice.

The older child who presents with an originally assigned sex of rearing that is inappropriate represents one of the most complex situations in clinical surgery. Raising a female pseudohermaphrodite as a male is one example. Care, extensive psychiatric and endocrinologic consultation, and real communication with the family are of utmost importance in these cases.

Surgical Management

Surgery continues to play a major role in the diagnosis of ambiguous genitalia, as only female pseudohermaphroditism can be diagnosed accurately by other means. With the increasing availability of hormone assays, some forms of male pseudohermaphroditism also will be diagnosed without the need for exploratory surgery, but this is still indicated in cases of true hermaphroditism, mixed gonadal dysgenesis, and many cases of male pseudohermaphroditism with confusion regarding gender assignment. Surgery is also necessary to remove inappropriate tissue and gonads with a high potential risk of neoplasm (the streak gonads with an XY karyotype).

Reconstructive surgery is required to feminize the external genitalia in female pseudohermaphrodites. This also is required with incompletely virilized male external genitalia. The management of hypospadias and cryptorchidism is not covered in this chapter.

Exploratory Surgery

Exploratory surgery involves gonadal biopsy, exploration to determine the nature of the internal ducts, and genital skin biopsy for fibroblast culture in cases of suspected androgen insensitivity. In addition, any endoscopic procedures that may clarify the nature of the abnormality and help in a more precise diagnosis should be performed at the same time. Laparoscopy can be useful at this stage of evaluation, allowing the determination of the nature of the internal ducts as well as the localization and biopsy of nonpalpable gonads when required. Gonadal biopsy is not indicated in female pseudohermaphroditism, which can be diagnosed accurately by other means.

Surgery Designed to Feminize the Partially Masculinized Patient

This surgery is designed to deal with three structures that have been partially or significantly masculinized in order to feminize them as appropriate for rearing in the female sex. These structures include the phallus (glans and corporal bodies), the labioscrotal folds, and the urogenital sinus. The exact anatomical diagnosis of the urogenital sinus must be made prior to planning any surgery. Currently, most of the reconstructive surgery is being done as a single procedure, but this depends on the level of entry of the vagina into the urogenital sinus. An exact understanding of the complexity of the abnormality is the most important factor in planning the type and timing of surgery. Virtually all of these patients will require clitoroplasty and reconstruction of the labioscrotal folds, which can be performed concurrently.[60, 61]

Patients with abnormal vaginal position must be investigated carefully by endoscopic and radiologic techniques to determine the exact anatomy prior to undertaking corrective procedures. In most patients with type I congenital adrenal hyperplasia, mixed gonadal dysgenesis, and true hermaphroditism, the vaginal opening is either in normal position or joining the urogenital sinus distally. In such cases, surgical reconstruction can be performed as a single-stage procedure that combines clitoroplasty, reconstruction of the labia minora, and posterior perineal (Fortunoff flap) reconstruction of the vaginal introitus. At this institution, this procedure is performed successfully within the first few months of life, although others prefer to wait until the infants are older.[62]

The technique that currently is most popular was described originally by

Allen in 1985 (Fig 8). This involves complete resection of the corporocavernosal bodies; partial resection of the glans (reduction plasty); meticulous preservation of the dorsal neurovascular bundle and ventral bridge of skin; and complete preservation of the phallic skin with Byar's-like flaps to re-create the labia minor simultaneously, as described by Perlmutter.[59] This is combined with a posterior-based, U-shaped flap in the vagina that joins the urogenital sinus in a low position.

In 1982, Allen et al. undertook a review of 42 patients at the Hospital of Sick Children in Toronto who had a variety of procedures encompassing these techniques. Satisfactory cosmetic results and normal postoperative clitoral sensation was present in all patients who had a reduction clitoroplasty and partial resection of the glans.[33] This surgery is best performed early in life to afford a cosmetic appearance consistent with the female sex of rearing, and to allay apprehension on the part of the parents and embarrassment with relatives.

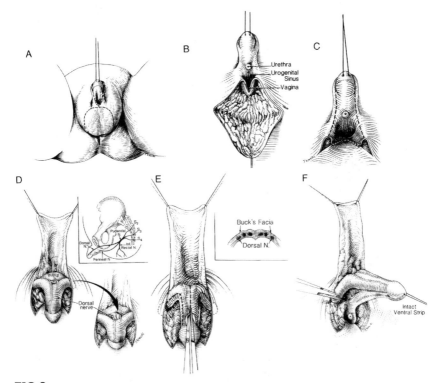

FIG 8.
Feminizing clitoroplasty and vaginoplasty, with preservation of neurovascular bundle and creation of labia minora. After making the initial incisions **(A)**, the urogenital sinus is divided along its posterior wall and extended 1 to 2 cm into the posterior wall of the vagina **(B)**. The perineal flap is then inlaid as a Y-V plasty to widen the introitus **(C)**. The corporal bodies are mobilized from the skin **(D)**, neurovascular bundles **(E)**, divided at the base **(F)**, separated from the glans **(G)**, then excised, with the glans fixed to the pubis **(H)**. *(Continued.)*

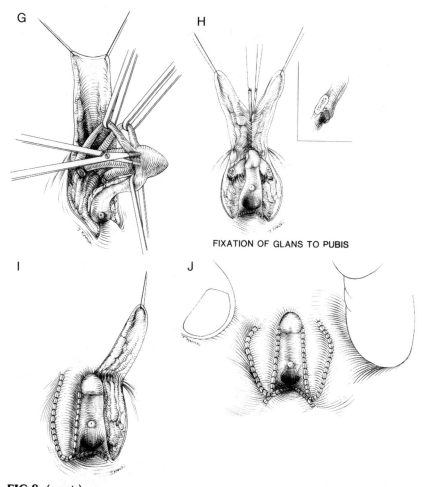

G

H

FIXATION OF GLANS TO PUBIS

I

J

FIG 8. (cont.).
The dorsal skin flap from the phallus is divided in the midline and sutured to the
coronal edge of the phallus and ventral skin flap to create labia minora **(I** and **J).**
(From Snyder HM, Retik AB, Bauer SB, et al: *J Urol* 1983; 129:1025–1026. Used
by permission.)

In those cases in which the vagina joins the urogenital sinus proximal to
the external sphincter, there is a significant increase in the complexity of
the surgery. As indicated previously, this must be diagnosed prior to planning any surgery. At the time of initial evaluation, in a small number of
children, the vaginal and urethral orifices will be confluent on the per-
ineum. Hendren has observed that in some of these cases, the vagina may
join the urethra proximal to the rhabdourinary sphincter. These children
constitute a small minority of the masculinized females, but it is imperative
to recognize this and avoid any further injury to the continence mecha-

nism. However, this may be deficient and require later bladder neck reconstruction. Hendren and Crawford[63] in the past advocated an extensive introital reconstruction utilizing a vaginal pull-down technique and perineal-based skin flaps. They noted the need for long-term vaginal dilatation using Hegar's dilators. To avoid this requirement for prolonged subsequent dilatation and, in some cases, surgical revision, a search has continued for a more cosmetically acceptable and functionally successful method of vaginoplasty for these cases. Two such options now exist. A recent publication by Passerini-Glazel[61] offers such an option. He described a transvesical approach to separate the vagina from the urethra, which can be accomplished under direct vision. The phallic skin then is tubularized along with a portion of the urethra. It is inverted and anastomosed under direct vision to the proximal vaginal stump (Figs 9 and 10). This procedure, although

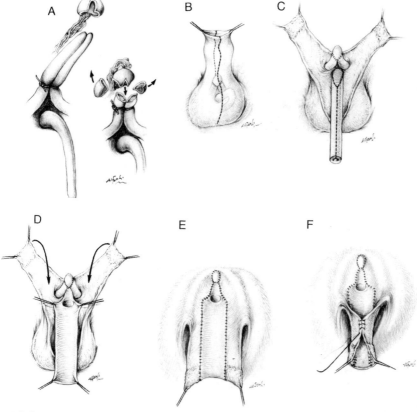

FIG 9.
Feminizing clitoroplasty, with preservation of neurovascular bundle and creation of neovagina from phallic skin and urethra **(A** and **B)**. The phallic portion of the urethra **(C)** is spatulated open **(D)** and sutured to the cutaneous flaps of the phallus **(E)**. These are then inverted to form a tube **(F)**. (Modified from Passerini-Glazel G: *J Urol* 1989; 142:566. Used by permission.)

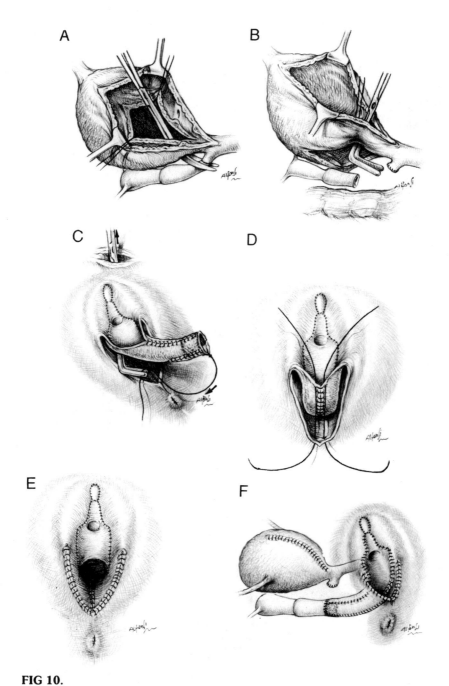

FIG 10.
Transtrigonal approach to the vagina inserting high into the urethra. The vagina is disconnected from the urethra **(A),** the stump is closed **(B),** and the neovagina is pulled through **(C)** and anastomosed **(D),** with completion of the introitus **(E** and **F).** (Modified from Passerini-Glazel G: *J Urol* 1989; 142:566. Used by permission.)

described in only four cases, has the advantage of interposing vascularized genital skin between the introital verge and the proximal vagina. In these cases, the surgical reconstruction is better performed at a later age, around 2 years. This also can be performed as a two-stage procedure with clitoral resection in early infancy, but in these cases, it does mean leaving the phallic skin at the time of the clitoral resection. Here also the phallic urethra is not available for incorporation into the vaginal tube.

A second option for the surgical repair of the high-entry vagina is the posterior sagittal approach advocated by Pena[64] and Hendren,[65] which may require simultaneous relocation or mobilization of the rectum. This is well described by Pena.[66]

At the time of puberty, a number of these children present requiring some form of vaginoplasty to allow normal menses and subsequent sexual intercourse. Many have had prior perineal surgery, and in such cases an extensive pull-through vaginoplasty may be required using inlay skin flaps or, if the latter are insufficient, full- or partial-thickness skin grafts, or the interposition of a segment of bowel. The use of Silastic prostheses is advocated to maintain patency of the newly created vagina in the postoperative period.

In summary, the establishment of an exact diagnosis in cases of ambiguous genitalia is critical. While all forms of intersex have aberrations of the normal endocrine control of phenotypic differentiation, in the neonatal period a prompt and complete diagnostic evaluation must be completed to determine the optimal sex of rearing. The potential for life-threatening electrolyte imbalance also must be recognized. The family crisis created in these situations requires support and diligent expertise in counseling and management. Specific therapy should be instituted promptly and very careful follow-up maintained.

References

1. Jost A: Problems of fetal endocrinology: The gonadal and hypophyseal hormones. *Recent Prog Horm Res* 1953; 8:379.
2. Jost A: Hormonal factors in the sex differentiation of the mammalian fetus. *Proc R Soc Lond [Biol]* 1970; 259:119.
3. Hamerton JL, Jacobs PA, Klinger HP: Paris Conference (1971): Standardization in human cytogenetics. *Birth Defects* 1972; 8:7.
4. Barr ML, Bertram EG: A morphological distinction between neurones of male and female, and the behaviour of the nucleolar satellite during acceleration of nucleoprotein synthesis. *Nature* 1949; 163:676.
5. WIlson JD, Goldstein JL: Classification of hereditary disorders of sexual development. *Birth Defects* 1975; 11:1–16.
6. Goodfellow PN: Mapping the Y chromosome. *Development* 1987; 101(suppl):39.
7. Page DC, Mosher R, Simpson EM, et al: The sex-determining region of the human Y chromosome encodes a finger protein. *Cell* 1987; 51:1091.
8. Mittwoch U: Males, females and hermaphrodites. *Ann Hum Genet* 1986; 50:103–121.

9. Eichwald EJ, Silmser CR: Communication. *Transplantation* 1955; 2:148.
10. Wolfe J: Other genes of the Y chromosome. *Development* 1987; 101(suppl): 117–118.
11. Burgoyne PS: The role of the mammalian Y chromosome in spermatogenesis. *Development* 1987; 101(suppl):133–141.
12. Byskov AG: Regulation of meiosis in mammals. Annales de Biologie Animale, Biochimie, Biophysique (Paris) 1979; 19:1251–1261.
13. Witschi E: Migration of the germ cells of human embryos from the yolksac to the primitive gonadal fold. *Contrib Embryology* 1948; 32:67–80.
14. Rogulska R, Ozdzenski W, Komar A: Behaviour of mouse primordial germ cells in the chick embryo. *J Embryol Exp Morphol* 1971; 25:115–164.
15. George FW, Wilson JD: Conversion of androgen to estrogen by the human fetal ovary. *J Clin Endocrinol Metab* 1978; 47:550.
16. Blanchard MG, Josso N: Source of the antiMullerian hormone synthesized by the fetal testis: Mullerian-inhibiting activity of the fetal bovine Sertoli-cells in tissue culture. *Pediatr Res* 1974; 8:968–971.
17. Donahoe PK, Ito Y, Price JM, et al: Mullerian-inhibiting substance activity in bovine fetal, newborn and prepubertal testes. *Biol Reprod* 1977; 16:238–243.
18. Picard JY, Josso N: Purification of testicular anti-mullerian hormone allowing direct visualization of the pure glycoprotein and determination of yield and purification factor. *Mol Cell Endocrinol* 1984; 34:23.
19. Picard JY, Benarous R, Guerrier D, et al: Cloning and expression of cDNA for anti-mullerian hormone. *Proc Natl Acad Sci U S A* 1986; 83:5464–5468.
20. Cohen-Haguenauer O, Picard JY, Mattei MG, et al: Mapping of the gene for anti-mullerian hormone to the short arm of human chromosome 19. *Cytogenet Cell Genet* 1987; 44:2.
21. Vigier B, Watrin F, Magre S, et al: Purified bovine AMH induces a characteristic freemartin effect in fetal rat prospective ovaries exposed to it in vitro. *Development* 1987; 100:43–55.
22. Vigier B, Forest MG, Eychenne B, et al: Anti-Mullerian hormone produces endocrine sex reversal of fetal ovaries. *Proc Natl Acad Sci U S A* 1989; 86:3684.
23. Tran D, Picard JY, Campargue J, et al: Immunocytochemical detection of anti mullerian hormone in Sertoli cells of various mammalian species including human. *J Histochem Cytochem* 1987; 35:733.
24. Wilson JD, Siiteri PK: Developmental pattern of testosterone synthesis in the fetal gonad of the rabbit. *Endocrinology* 1973; 92:1182–1191.
25. Wilson JD: Sexual differentiation. *Annu Rev Physiol* 1978; 40:279–306.
26. Meyer WJ, Migeon BR, Migeon CJ: Locus on human X chromosome for dihydrotestosterone receptor and androgen insensitivity. *Proc Natl Acad Sci U S A* 1975; 72:1469.
27. Gruenwald P: The relation of the growing mullerian duct to the wolffian duct and its importance for the genesis of malformation. *Anat Rec* 1941; 81:1–15.
28. Glenister TW: The development of the utricle and of the so-called middle lobe or median lobe of the human prostate. *J Anat* 1962; 96:443–447.
29. Grumbach MM, Conte FA: Disorders of sex differentiation, in Williams RH (ed): *Textbook of Endocrinology*. Philadelphia, WB Saunders Co, 1981, pp 423–513.
30. Hamilton WJ, Mossman HW: The urogenital system, in *Human Embryology: Prenatal Development of Form and Function,* ed 4. New York, The Macmillan Press, 1976.

31. Kellklumpu-Lehtinen P: Development of sexual dimorphism in human urogenital sinus complex. *Biol Neonate* 1985; 48:157.
32. Allen T: Disorders of sexual differentiation. *Urology* 1976; 7:1–32.
33. Allen LE, Hardy BE, Churchill BM: The surgical management of enlarged clitoris. *J Urol* 1982; 128:351–354.
34. Conte FA, Grumbach MM: Abnormalities of sexual differentiation, in Smith DR (ed): *General Urology.* Los Altos, California, Lange Medical Publications, 1984; pp 574–597.
35. Allen T: Disorders of sexual differentiation, in Kelalis PP, King LR, Belman AB (eds): *Clinical Pediatric Urology,* ed 2. Philadelphia, WB Saunders Co, 1985, pp 904–921.
36. Zachman M, Werber EA, Prader A: Two types of male pseudohermaphroditism due to 17-20 desmolase deficiency. *J Clin Endocrinol Metab* 1982; 55:487.
37. Larrea F, Lisker R, Banuelos R, et al: Hypergonadotrophic hypogonadism in a XX female subject due to 17-20 steroid desmolase deficiency. *Acta Endocrinol (Copenh)* 1983; 103:400.
38. Brown TR, Maes M, Rothwell SW, et al: Human complete androgen insensitivity with normal DHT receptor binding capacity in cultures of genital skin fibroblasts: Evidence for a qualitative abnormality of the receptor. *J Clin Endocrinol Metab* 1982; 55:61–68.
39. Griffin JE, Wilson JD: The syndromes of androgen resistance. *N Engl J Med* 1980; 320:198–209.
40. Imperato-McGinley J, Guerrero L, Gauthier T, et al: Steroid 5α-reductase deficiency in men: An inherited form of male pseudohermaphroditism. *Science* 1974; 186:1213.
41. Imperato-McGinley J, Gauthier T, Pichardo M, et al: The diagnosis of 5α-reductase deficiency in infancy. *J Clin Endocrinol Metab* 1986; 63:1313–1318.
42. Lorge F, Wese FX, Sluysmans T, et al: L'ambiguité sexuelle: Aspects urologiques. *Acta Urol Belg* 1989; 57:647–661.
43. Hughes IA, Evans BAJ: The fibroblast as a model for androgen resistant states. *J Clin Endocrinol Metab* 1988; 28:565–579.
44. Klinefelter HF Jr, Reinstein EC Jr, Albright F: Syndrome characterized by gynecomastia, aspermatogenesis without A-Leydigism, and increased excretion of follicle stimulating hormone. *J Clin Endocrinol Metab* 1942; 2:615.
45. Leonard JM, Paulsen CA, Ospina LF, et al: The classification of Klinefelter's syndrome, in Vallet HL, Porter IH (eds): *Genetic Mechanisms of Sexual Development.* New York, Academic Press, 1979, pp 407–423.
46. Guerrier D, Tran D, Van der Winden JM, et al: The persisting Mullerian duct syndrome: A molecular approach. *J Clin Endocrinol Metab* 1989; 68:46–52.
47. Page D, de la Chapelle A: The parental origin of X chromosome in XX males determined using restriction fragment length polymorphisms. *Am J Hum Genet* 1984; 36:565.
48. Magenis RE, Casanova M, Fellous M, et al: Further cytological evidence for Xp-Yp translocation in XX males using in situ hybridization with Y-derived probe. *Hum Genet* 1987; 75:228–233.
49. Petit C, de la Chapelle A, Levilliers J, et al: An abnormal terminal X-Y interchange accounts for most but not all cases of human XX maleness. *Cell* 1987; 49:595–602.
50. Lalau-Keraly J, Amice V, Chaussain JL, et al: L'hermaphrodisme vrai. *Ann Pediatr* (Paris) 1986; 33:87–91.

51. Luks FI, Hansbrough F, Klotz DH Jr, et al: Early gender assignment in true hermaphroditism. *J Pediatr Surg* 1988; 23:1122.
52. Mayou BG, Armon P, Linderbaum RH: Pregnancy and childbirth in true hermaphrodite following reconstructive surgery. *Br J Obstet Gynaecol* 1978; 85:314–316.
53. Tegenkamp TR, Brazzell JW, Tegenkamp I, et al: Pregnancy without benefit of reconstructive surgery in a bisexually active true hermaphrodite. *Am J Obstet Gynecol* 1979; 135:427–428.
54. Narita O, Manba S, Nakanishi T, et al: Pregnancy and childbirth in a true hermaphrodite. *Obstet Gynecol* 12975; 45:593.
55. Van Niekerk WA: True hermaphroditism. *Pediatr Adolesc Endocrinol* 1981; 8:80.
56. Behesti M, Churchill BM, Hardy BE, et al: Familial persistent Mullerian duct syndrome. *J Urol* 1983; 131:968–969.
57. Hughes IA, Davies PAD: Neonatal endocrine and metabolic emergencies. *J Clin Endocrinol Metab* 1980; 9:583–604.
58. Feldman KW, Smith DW: Fetal phallic growth and penile standards for newborn male infants. *J Pediatr* 1975; 86:395.
59. Perlmutter AD: Management of intersexuality, in *Campbell's Urology*, vol 2, ed 4. Philadelphia, WB Saunders Co, 1979, p 1535.
60. Donahoe PK: The diagnosis and treatment of infants with intersex abnormalities. *Pediatr Clin North Am* 1987; 34:1333–1348.
61. Passerini-Glazel G: A new technique for vaginal reconstruction in severely masculinized female pseudohermaphrodites. *J Urol* 1989; 142:565–568.
62. Churchill BM, McLorie GA: Intersex, in Gillenwater JY, Grayhack JT, Howards SS, et al (eds): *Adult and Pediatric Urology*. Chicago, Year Book Medical Publishers, 1987, pp 1916–1931.
63. Hendren WH, Crawford JD: Adrenogenital syndrome: The anatomy of the anomaly and its repair: Some new concepts. *J Pediatr Surg* 1969; 4:49.
64. Pena A: The surgical management of persistent cloaca: Results in 54 patients treated with a posterior sagittal approach. *J Pediatr Surg* 1989; 24:590–598.
65. Hendren WH: Repair of cloacal anomalies: Current techniques. *J Pediatr Surg* 1986; 12:1159–1176.
66. Pena A: *An Atlas: Surgical Management of Anorectal Malformations*. New York, Springer-Verlag, 1990.

Index

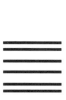

BUSINESS REPLY MAIL

FIRST CLASS   PERMIT No. 135   ST. LOUIS, MO.

POSTAGE WILL BE PAID BY ADDRESSEE

PAT NEWMAN
Mosby-Year Book, Inc.
11830 Westline Industrial Drive
P.O. Box 46908
St. Louis, Missouri 63146-9988

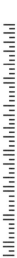

FREE Examination Privileges

Yes! I'd like to review a new Year Book. Please send me a FREE 30-day examination copy of the book(s) checked below:

[ ] Year Book of **Anesthesia** (22137)	$57.95
[ ] Year Book of **Cardiology** (22114)	$57.95
[ ] Year Book of **Critical Care Medicine** (22091)	$54.95
[ ] Year Book of **Dermatology** (22108)	$57.95
[ ] Year Book of **Diagnostic Radiology** (22132)	$57.95
[ ] Year Book of **Digestive Diseases** (22081)	$57.95
[ ] Year Book of **Drug Therapy** (22139)	$57.95
[ ] Year Book of **Emergency Medicine** (22085)	$57.95
[ ] Year Book of **Endocrinology** (22107)	$57.95
[ ] Year Book of **Family Practice** (20801)	$54.95
[ ] Year Book of **Geriatrics and Gerontology** (22121)	$54.95
[ ] Year Book of **Hand Surgery** (22096)	$57.95
[ ] Year Book of **Hematology** (20418)	$54.95
[ ] Year Book of **Health Care Management** (21145)	$54.95
[ ] Year Book of **Infectious Diseases** (20420)	$54.95
[ ] Year Book of **Infertility** (20414)	$54.95
[ ] Year Book of **Medicine** (22087)	$57.95
[ ] Year Book of **Neonatal-Perinatal Medicine** (22117)	$54.95
[ ] Year Book of **Neurology and Neurosurgery** (22120)	$57.95
[ ] Year Book of **Nuclear Medicine** (22140)	$57.95
[ ] Year Book of **Obstetrics and Gynecology** (22118)	$57.95
[ ] Year Book of **Occupational and Environmental Medicine** (22092)	$57.95
[ ] Year Book of **Oncology** (20415)	$54.95
[ ] Year Book of **Ophthalmology** (22135)	$57.95
[ ] Year Book of **Orthopedics** (20417)	$54.95
[ ] Year Book of **Otolaryngology – Head and Neck Surgery** (22086)	$57.95
[ ] Year Book of **Pathology and Clinical Pathology** (22104)	$57.95
[ ] Year Book of **Pediatrics** (22088)	$54.95
[ ] Year Book of **Plastic and Reconstructive Surgery** (22112)	$57.95
[ ] Year Book of **Psychiatry and Applied Mental Health** (22110)	$57.95
[ ] Year Book of **Pulmonary Disease** (22109)	$54.95
[ ] Year Book of **Speech Language and Hearing** (21144)	$59.95
[ ] Year Book of **Sports Medicine** (20419)	$54.95
[ ] Year Book of **Surgery** (22084)	$57.95
[ ] Year Book of **Ultrasound** (21170)	$75.00
[ ] Year Book of **Urology** (20416)	$54.95
[ ] Year Book of **Vascular Surgery** (22105)	$57.95

*All Year Books are published annually. For your convenience, we will add your name to our subscriber list and send you an announcement of each future volume about 2 months before publication. The new volume will be shipped to you unless you complete and return the cancellation notice enclosed with the announcement and we receive it within the time indicated. Don't forget, you may cancel your subscription at any time. The Year Book is yours FREE for 30 days, and may be returned for full credit. Return postage is guaranteed.

NAME/ACCT. NO.

ADDRESS

CITY/STATE/ZIP

Prepaid orders are shipped postage free; add $3.50 per order to cover handling. Other orders will be billed a shipping and handling charge. Please add applicable sales tax. Prices quoted in U.S. dollars. Canadian orders will be billed in U.S. funds. All prices subject to change without notice.

Mosby-Year Book, Inc. • 11830 Westline Industrial Drive • St. Louis, MO 63146

MC-0277